D0023512

Atlas of
EPILEPSY

Atlas of
EPILEPSY
Second Edition

Richard E Appleton MA FRCP

Roald Dahl EEG Unit
Alder Hey Children's Hospital
Liverpool, UK

Andrew Nicolson MD MRCP

The Walton Centre for
Neurology & Neurosurgery
Liverpool, UK

David W Chadwick
DM FRCP

The Walton Centre for
Neurology & Neurosurgery
Liverpool, UK

James M MacKenzie
MBChB(Ed) FRCPath

Department of Pathology
Medical School
Foresterhill
Aberdeen Royal Hospital Trust
Aberdeen, UK

David F Smith
MD MRCP

The Walton Centre for
Neurology & Neurosurgery
Liverpool, UK

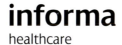

© 2007 Informa UK Ltd

First published in the United Kingdom in 1998 by Parthenon Publishing
Second edition published in 2007 by Informa Healthcare, 4 Park Square, Milton Park, Abingdon, Oxon OX14 4RN.
Informa Healthcare is a trading division of Informa UK Ltd. Registered Office: 37/41 Mortimer Street, London W1T 3JH.
Registered in England and Wales Number 1072954.

Tel.: +44 (0)20 7017 6000
Fax: +44 (0)20 7017 6699
E-mail: info.medicine@tandf.co.uk
Website: www.informahealthcare.com

Second printing 2007

All rights reserved. No part of this publication may be reproduced, stored in a retrieval system, or transmitted, in any form or by any means, electronic, mechanical, photocopying, recording, or otherwise, without the prior permission of the publisher or in accordance with the provisions of the Copyright, Designs and Patents Act 1988 or under the terms of any licence permitting limited copying issued by the Copyright Licensing Agency, 90 Tottenham Court Road, London W1P 0LP.

Although every effort has been made to ensure that all owners of copyright material have been acknowledged in this publication, we would be glad to acknowledge in subsequent reprints or editions any omissions brought to our attention.

A CIP record for this book is available from the British Library.

Library of Congress Cataloging-in-Publication Data

Data available on application

ISBN10: 1-84214-027-2
ISBN13: 978-1-84214-027-7

Distributed in North and South America by

Taylor & Francis
6000 Broken Sound Parkway, NW, (Suite 300)
Boca Raton, FL 33487, USA

Within Continental USA
Tel.: 1(800)272 7737; Fax: 1(800)374 3401
Outside Continental USA
Tel.: (561)994 0555; Fax: (561)361 6018
E-mail: orders@crcpress.com

Distributed in the rest of the world by
Thomson Publishing Services
Cheriton House
North Way
Andover, Hampshire SP10 5BE, UK
Tel.: +44 (0)1264 332424
E-mail: tps.tandfsalesorder@thomson.com

Composition by Parthenon Publishing

Printed and bound in India by Replika Press Pvt. Ltd.

Contents

Preface

Epilepsy is much more than a functional disorder of the central nervous system as described by Hughlings Jackson over almost a century and a half ago as 'the expression of occasional, sudden, excessive, rapid local discharges in the grey matter'; it has evolved and has been transformed into a dramatic and vivid series of visual images. More appropriately, the epilepsies are now regarded as a collection of conditions with different pathophysiologies, multiple manifestations and diverse etiologies – yet it still remains one of the most poorly understood groups of conditions that affect human kind.

There is a tremendous amount of information regarding the epidemiology, natural history and prognosis of the epilepsies, much of which can be illustrated simply, but effectively, in graphic form. The increasing technological sophistication and understanding of the basic mechanisms and causes of epileptic seizures emphasize the importance of the visual aspects of epilepsy.

The electroencephalogram (EEG), which allows the pictorial display of abnormal cerebral activity, is central to the classification of the epilepsies and epilepsy syndromes. Computed tomography and magnetic resonance imaging have revealed not only the obvious, but also the many subtle, structural abnormalities in the brain responsible for seizures, as well as their susceptibility to surgical treatment. Advances in single-photon computed emission tomography and positron emission tomography have allowed the production of 'functional' images of the brain that are particularly relevant to epileptogenesis and the latest advances in functional magnetic resonance imaging are now able to highlight specific fibers and tracts of fibers (and their networks) that may be involved in both the onset and propagation of individual seizures.

The treatment of epilepsy has, since the time of Hughlings Jackson, improved dramatically with the advent of more effective and less toxic antiepileptic drugs, and the development of specialist interdisciplinary services. More specifically, surgical ablation of epileptic foci has vividly demonstrated the marked neuropathological heterogeneity of the epilepsies. In contrast to ablative or destructive procedures, the last decade has seen surgical attention focusing on stimulation techniques to improve seizure-control, including vagal nerve and deep brain stimulation.

The first edition of *Atlas of Epilepsy* provided a unique pictorial representation of and perspective on, the most common group of disorders of the central nervous system. The second edition of *Atlas of Epilepsy* contains new and updated text, Figures and Tables to reflect the further advances that have been made in the knowledge and understanding of the epilepsies over the past decade. This new edition with its dramatic representation of epilepsy should continue to be of interest and value to all those who are involved with the subject.

Richard E Appleton
Andrew Nicolson
David W Chadwick
James M MacKenzie
David F Smith

Liverpool and Aberdeen

Acknowledgments

The authors would like to thank the following individuals for their invaluable help and contributions to this project:

Mrs S Schofield, Mrs M Beirne, Mrs B Acomb and Ms L Beeston, The Roald Dahl EEG Unit, Royal Liverpool Children's Hospital, Alder Hey, Liverpool; Dr L Abernethy and Professor H Carty, Consultant Pediatric Radiologists, Royal Liverpool Children's Hospital, Alder Hey, Liverpool; Professor J Stephenson, Consultant Pediatric Neurologist, Royal Hospital for Sick Children, Glasgow; Dr CP Panayiotopoulos, Consultant in Clinical Neurophysiology, St Thomas' Hospital, London; Drs K Das, S Niven, TE Nixon and ET Smith, Consultant Neuroradiologists, Walton Centre for Neurology and Neurosurgery, Liverpool; Dr TH Turnbull, Consultant Neuroradiologist, Hope Hospital, Salford; Professor J Duncan, Consultant Neurologist, National Hospital for Neurology and Neurosurgery, London; Professor M Pirmohamed, Royal Liverpool University Hospital; Dr R Duncan, Consultant Neurologist, Southern General Hospital, Glasgow; Mr T Lesser, Consultant ENT Surgeon, Aintree Hospital NHS Trust, Liverpool; and Dr H Cross, Institute of Child Health and Great Ormond Street Hospital for Children NHS Trust, London.

1. Definitions and basic mechanisms

DEFINITIONS

Seizures and epilepsy are clinical phenomena resulting from hyperexcitability of the neurons of the cerebral hemispheres. They may be defined in both physiological and clinical terms.

> *Physiologically*, epilepsy is the name for occasional sudden, excessive, rapid and local discharges of gray matter. Evidence to date indicates that increased and hypersynchronous neuronal discharges are the essential features involved in the generation of seizures.

> *Clinically*, an epileptic seizure is an intermittent stereotypical, usually unprovoked, disturbance of consciousness, behavior, emotion, motor function or sensation that is the result of cortical neuronal discharge. Epilepsy is a condition in which seizures recur, usually spontaneously.

BASIC MECHANISMS OF EPILEPSY

There are fundamental physiological differences between focal and generalized epileptogenesis, which probably explain their wide range of clinical manifestations and varied responses to different antiepileptic agents.

Focal epileptogenesis

The cellular correlate of the interictal spike wave is a paroxysmal depolarization shift (PDS) of the resting membrane potential, which triggers a brief rapid burst of action potentials terminated by a sustained after-hyperpolarization (Figure 1.1). The PDS may be the result either of an imbalance between excitatory (glutamate and aspartate) and inhibitory (gamma-aminobutyric acid; GABA) neurotransmitters or of abnormalities of voltage-controlled membrane ion channels. Increased sodium and calcium conductance, and reduced potassium conductance favor depolarization and burst firing.

Asynchronous burst-firing occurs spontaneously in some hippocampal and cortical neurons. Synchronization of neuronal burst behavior and propagation of epileptic discharges require both impaired inhibition and intact excitatory synaptic connections. The initiation of focal epileptogenesis is probably due to an imbalance between endogenous neuromodulators, with acetylcholine favoring depolarization and dopamine enhancing neuronal membrane stability.

Knowledge of the structure of neurotransmitter receptors provides a means of understanding the modes of action of conventional antiepileptic drugs and serves as a basis for the rational development of new antiepileptic agents.

$GABA_A$ receptor and chloride ion channel

GABA is the major inhibitory neurotransmitter in the central nervous system. There is compelling evidence that loss of postsynaptic GABA-mediated inhibition is crucial to the genesis of focal seizures.

Activation of the $GABA_A$ receptor (Figure 1.2) opens the chloride channel on the GABA/benzodiazepine complex, allowing chloride influx, hyperpolarization of the postsynaptic neuron and inhibition of firing. Several antiepileptic drugs (and experimental compounds) exert their antiepileptic effects via mechanisms which enhance GABA-mediated inhibition (Table 1.1). Vigabatrin, a suicidal inhibitor of GABA transaminase, was the first antiepileptic drug to be developed with a specific mode of action.

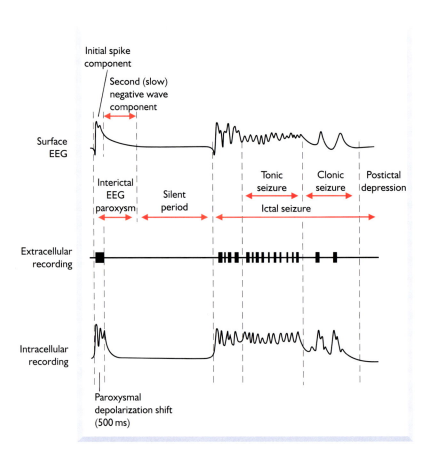

Figure 1.1 Schematic representation of neurophysiological events in seizure disorders. With permission from reference 1

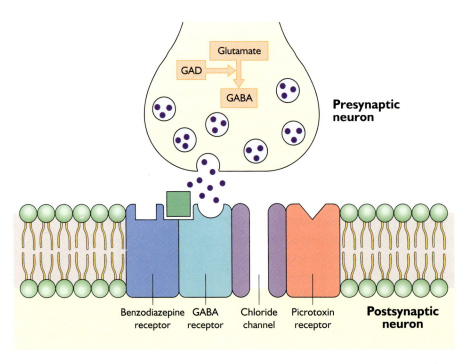

Figure 1.2 GABA receptor, chloride–ionophore complex and benzodiazepine receptor complex. GABA, gamma-aminobutyric acid; GAD, glutamic acid decarboxylase

NMDA receptor and calcium channel

Glutamate is the predominant excitatory neurotransmitter in the nervous system. Four postsynaptic receptor subtypes can be identified, according to preferential binding of endogenous ligands.

The N-methyl-D-aspartate (NMDA) receptor (Figure 1.3) is most likely to have a role in epilepsy. Stimulation of this receptor produces an intracellular cationic flux, particularly calcium, with rapid depolarization and sustained repetitive firing. NMDA antagonists are potent anticonvulsants in animal models, but their clinical evaluation has been limited by neurotoxicity.

Table 1.1 Pharmacological enhancement of GABA-mediated inhibition

Mechanism	Compound
True GABA agonist	
GABA$_A$ receptor	muscimol
GABA$_B$ receptor	baclofen
GABA prodrug	progabide
Stimulation of GABA synthesis	milacemide
Allosteric enhancement of GABA efficacy	benzodiazepines anticonvulsant beta-carbolines
Direct action on chloride ionophore	phenobarbitone
Inhibition of GABA re-uptake	nipecotic acid tiagabine
Inhibition of GABA transaminase	vigabatrin

Table 1.2 Pharmacological approaches to decrease glutamatergic neurotransmission

Mechanism	Compound
Decreased glutamate synthesis (glutaminase inhibitors)	aserazine
Decreased presynaptic glutamate release	adenosine analog lamotrigine
Postsynaptic receptor antagonists	
non-selective	kynurenic acid topiramate
selective NMDA antagonists	
competitive	CPP
non-competitive	MK801 remacemide
kainate/quisqualate antagonists metabotropic receptor antagonists	
Enhanced glutamate uptake	
Long-term downregulation of the excitatory amino acid (EAA) system	

CPP, 3-[(*)-2-carboxy-piperazin-4-yl]propyl-1-phosphonate

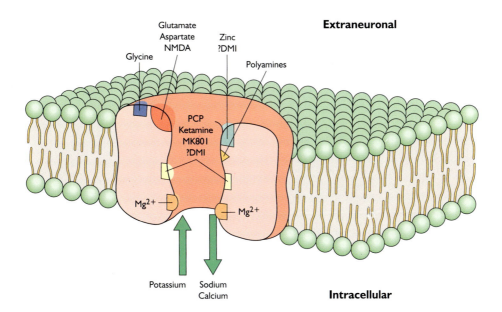

Figure 1.3 NMDA receptor-operated ion channel showing the variety of binding sites. DMI, desmethylimipramine; PCP, phencyclidine; Zn, zinc; Mg, magnesium

However, excitatory neurotransmission can be manipulated in other ways (Table 1.2). The novel antiepileptic drug lamotrigine acts via inhibition of the release of glutamate presynaptically.

Voltage-sensitive sodium channels

A number of conventional (phenytoin and carbamazepine) and novel antiepileptic drugs (lamotrigine) act by voltage-dependent modulation of sodium channels. This involves a shift in steady-state inactivation to hyperpolarized membrane voltages. This shift has been experimentally demonstrated for both phenytoin and lamotrigine. Consequently, drug-bound inactivated sodium channels cannot easily return to the resting state, thereby preventing conduction of sodium, depolarization and sustained repetitive firing.

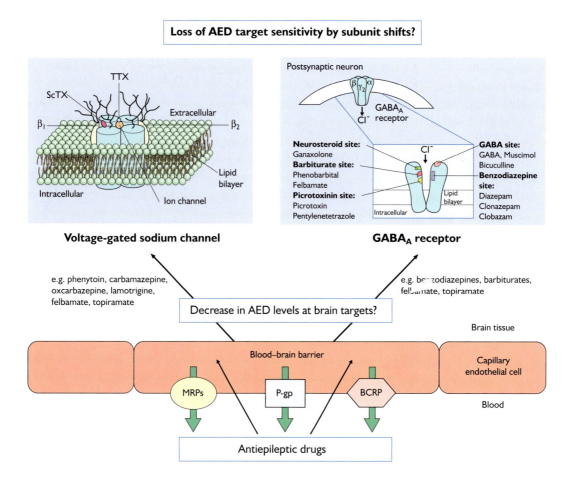

Figure 1.4 Schematic illustration of the multidrug transporter and drug target hypotheses of drug resistance in epilepsy. In order to reach their targets in the brain, antiepileptic drugs (AEDs) must penetrate through the blood–brain barrier, which is formed by capillary endothelial cells as illustrated in the figure. Numerous drug efflux transporters are located at the luminal (blood-directed) membrane of these cells, aiming to protect the brain from intoxication by lipophilic xenobiotics, including numerous drugs, which otherwise would penetrate from the blood into the brain by passive diffusion, without limitation. These efflux transporters include P-glycoprotein (P-gp), multidrug resistance proteins (MRPs) and breast cancer-related protein (BCRP). These transporters are locally over-expressed in epileptogenic tissue, thereby reducing the amount of AEDs that reaches the brain targets. Apart from this transporter-based loss of efficacy, AEDs may lose efficacy because of alterations in brain targets, including ion channels or neurotransmitter receptors. As shown in the figure, most AEDs act by either modulating voltage-gated sodium channels or GABA_A receptor-associated chloride channels[3]. The subunit composition and/or expression of sodium channels and GABA_A receptors seem to change in epileptogenic tissue, thereby leading to alterations in the efficacy of many AEDs that act via these targets[2]. With permission from reference 4

Generalized epileptogenesis

The generalized spike-and-wave (GSW) seizure is produced by an abnormal thalamocortical interaction which oscillates between enhanced excitation with firing (spike wave) and enhanced inhibition with hyperpolarization (slow wave). In humans, the primary abnormality is cortical hyperexcitability, which may be due to a genetically determined metabolic defect or a minor morphological abnormality such as microdysgenesis.

There is strong evidence that generalized epileptogenesis is mediated via calcium T channels, which are found in high density in thalamic neurons and activated by relatively low-voltage thresholds after sustained depolarization. The resultant low-threshold calcium current (LTCC) generates a low-threshold calcium spike (LTCS), which underlies the slow thalamic rhythms seen in 3-cycles per second (cps) GSW or absence seizures. The selective blockade of calcium T channels is the likely mechanism of action of antiabsence drugs such as ethosuximide.

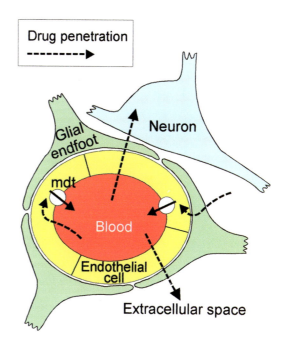

Figure 1.5 Schematic representation of the blood–brain barrier and drug transport. With permission from reference 5

PHARMACOGENETICS (DRUG RESPONSIVENESS AND DRUG RESISTANCE)

There is considerable research into, and excitement about, the mechanism of responsiveness and resistance to antiepileptic drugs – the phenomenon of pharmacogenetics (or pharmacogenomics) – that might explain why individuals with the same electroclinical epilepsy syndrome or identical seizure types may respond in completely different ways to the same drug[2] (Figure 1.4). The reasons for this apparent resistance are likely to be multifactorial but two hypotheses supported by clinical and experimental data include:

(1) Removal of the antiepileptic drugs from neural (including the specific epileptogenic) tissue through excessive expression (and overactivity) of drug transporter proteins (Figure 1.5);

(2) Reduced or even absent drug-target sensitivity in epileptogenic brain tissue.

Research is ongoing to confirm or refute these hypotheses (or to identify other potential mechanisms), and it is possible that results from this work may also clarify why seizure control is never regained in the very small (but clinically important) group of patients who relapse when antiepileptic medication is withdrawn having been initially seizure free for 2 or more years. Finally, it is tempting – but probably naively optimistic – to hope that this may also lead to a reduction in, or even prevention of, drug-resistance.

REFERENCES

1. Ayala GF, Matsumoto H, Gumnit RJ. Excitability changes and inhibitory mechanisms in neocortical neurones during seizures. J Neurophysiol 1970; 33: 73–85

2. Schmidt D, Loscher W. Drug resistance in epilepsy: putative neurobiologic and clinical mechanisms. Epilepsia 2005; 46: 858–77

3. Rogawski MA, Löscher W. The neurobiology of antiepileptic drugs. Nat Rev Neurosci 2004; 5: 553–64

4. Löscher W. Mechanisms of drug resistance. Epileptic Disord 2005; 7 (Suppl 1): 53–9

5. Löscher W, Potschka H. Role of multidrug transporters in pharmacoresistance to antiepileptic drugs. J Pharmacol Exp Ther 2002; 301: 7–14

2.   Epidemiology

Epilepsy is the most common of the neurological disorders. The most complete epidemiological study, from Rochester, Minnesota, reports an age- and gender-adjusted annual incidence of 49 per 100 000 population, with peaks both in the first year of life and in senescence, and a lifetime cumulative incidence of 3% by age 80 years (Figure 2.1).

The most recent data define a prevalence of 6.8/1000 population, which suggests that approximately 400 000 (60–70 000 in persons < 16 years of age) subjects in the UK and 2 000 000 in the USA have active epilepsy. The large and ever-increasing gap between point prevalence and lifetime cumulative incidence is a reflection, in many cases, of the self-limiting nature of the condition. Approximately one-third of all epilepsies that have an onset in childhood will spontaneously remit by early adult life. The chance of a spontaneous remission will depend largely on the specific epilepsy syndrome.

The age-adjusted annual death rate for epilepsy varies widely among countries (0.4–4/100 000), perhaps due to differences in prevalence rates and/or different methods of recording on death certificates. The factors associated with a higher mortality include male gender, age (< 1 year, > 50 years), marital status (single) and epilepsy symptomatic of diffuse or focal cerebral disease.

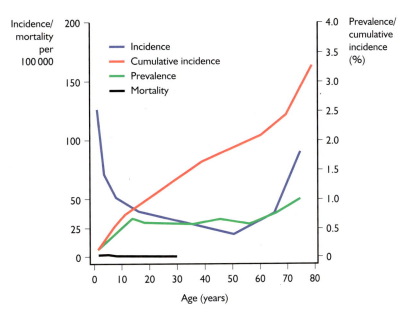

Figure 2.1 Incidence and cumulative incidence, prevalence and mortality rates for epilepsy in Rochester, Minnesota (1935–1974) study. With permission from reference 1

Table 2.1 Standardized mortality ratios for patients with epilepsy in the Rochester study (1935–1974) by etiology of the epilepsy and follow-up period. With permission from reference 2

Years of follow-up	Total	Idiopathic	Neurodeficit since birth	Potentially acquired secondary epilepsy
0–1	3.8	2.5	20.0	4.3
2–4	2.4	1.7	33.3	2.0
5–9	2.0	2.4	2.0	1.6
10–19	1.4	1.1	6.7	1.1
20–29	2.4	2.0	10.0	3.3
Total	2.3	1.8	11.0	2.2

The standardized mortality ratio for epilepsy is high (Table 2.1). In approximately 25% of cases, death may be related to seizures (status epilepticus, accidental injury and sudden unexplained death). Suicide and cerebral tumors are over-represented as causes of death in patients with epilepsy.

Sudden Unexplained Death in Epilepsy (SUDEP) has been (and continues to be) the focus of numerous research and epidemiological studies over the past decade. One important case-controlled study on SUDEP reported that people who had not been seizure free in the previous year had a 23-fold increased risk of SUDEP, compared with people with fully controlled seizures and the risks increased with increasing seizure frequency[3]. As a consequence of this interest, the Department of Health in the UK sponsored a National Sentinel Clinical Audit of epilepsy-related deaths, published in 2002, which identified a number of predestined but potentially avoidable and preventable factors that might be implicated in a greater risk of death in children and adults with epilepsy[4]. SUDEP appears to be less common in children than in adults and is more commonly seen in children with symptomatic epilepsy and with additional physical and/or learning difficulties, where there is an approximately 20-fold increased risk of dying compared with children with an idiopathic epilepsy and without additional physical and/or learning difficulties[5,6].

REFERENCES

1. Anderson VE, Hauser WA, Rich S. Genetic heterogeneity in the epilepsies. Adv Neurol 1986; 44: 59–75

2. Hauser WA, Annegers JF, Elveback LR. Mortality in patients with epilepsy. Epilepsia 1980; 21: 399–412

3. Nilsson L, Farahmand BY, Persson P-G, et al. Risk factors for sudden unexplained death in epilepsy: a case-control study. Lancet 1999; 353: 888–93

4. Hanna NJ, Black, M, Sander JWS, et al. The National Sentinel Clinical Audit of Epilepsy-Related Death: Epilepsy – Death in the Shadows. 2002. London: The Stationery Office

5. Gordon N. Sudden unexpected death in epilepsy. Dev Med Child Neurol 2001; 43: 354–7

6. Appleton RE. Mortality in paediatric epilepsy. Arch Dis Child 2004; 88: 1091–4

3.   Diagnosis

Epilepsy is a symptom of a disorder of the cerebral hemispheres with a diverse etiology. A complete diagnosis of epilepsy is a four-step process: differentiation of seizures from other causes of altered consciousness or behavior; differentiation of spontaneous unprovoked seizures from acute symptomatic seizures; classification of seizures and epilepsy syndrome; and determination of the underlying cause. An additional step in establishing as comprehensive a diagnosis as possible is to consider any additional neurological (physical or cognitive) features or impairment.

DIFFERENTIAL DIAGNOSIS

Differentiation of seizures from other paroxysmal disorders with or without loss of consciousness can usually be achieved on clinical grounds alone, but may be difficult in some cases, particularly in young children.

The patient's history should include a detailed account of the symptoms before, during (if consciousness retained) and after the event(s) as well as the circumstances surrounding the attacks and, in particular, a clear eye-witness description. If diagnostic doubt remains, a policy of 'wait-and-see' should be adopted, as the diagnosis will usually be revealed by further events. Patients (or their parents if appropriate) should be asked to make a record, in written detail, of all further episodes and to present this information at subsequent reviews.

The use of a videocamera may be extremely useful in diagnosing epileptic vs. non-epileptic paroxysmal events and may compensate for inadequate or inaccurate histories from eye-witnesses. In addition, on occasions, recording the symptomatic events with continuous ambulatory electroencephalography (EEG) or inpatient video-EEG telemetry monitoring will allow the differentiation of epileptic from non-epileptic attacks.

Neonatal seizures may be both over- and under-diagnosed. Generalized tonic-clonic seizures do not occur in neonates, in whom most seizures are localized (focal), fragmentary clonic, tonic or myoclonic. Many seizures are subtle and consist only of abnormal movement patterns such as mouthing/chewing, bicycling or boxing, or apnea and, thus, may easily go unrecognized.

Not all abnormal movements are seizures. The resultant difficulty in seizure recognition is greatest in premature infants. EEG recordings (specifically with simultaneous video recording of clinical events) may resolve some of the difficulty, but there still remains the problem of 'electroclinical dissociation' in that electroencephalographically recognized seizures have an uncertain and inconstant relationship with clinical seizures.

Finally, a diagnosis of epilepsy in a child should be confirmed by a hospital clinician – a pediatrician, pediatric neurologist or adult neurologist – before investigations are performed or treatment initiated. The risk of a child with epilepsy coming to harm from a delay in diagnosis is minimal compared with the considerable potential and genuine harm that may arise from a false-positive diagnosis.

The differential diagnoses of epilepsy in children and in adults are summarized in Tables 3.1 and 3.2, respectively.

In children, simple faints (with or without brief hypoxic myoclonic or clonic seizures), migraine, night terrors, sleep myoclonus, cardiac arrhythmias

Table 3.1 Differential diagnosis of epilepsy in children

Episodes with altered consciousness	Episodes without altered consciousness
Delirium (with any febrile illness)	tics, rhythmic motor habits or mannerisms
Syncope (simple faint)	shuddering spells
Cyanotic ('blue') breath-holding attacks	rigors (with any febrile illness)
Pallid syncopal attacks (reflex anoxic seizures)	jitteriness (newborn period)
Night terrors	hypnagogic jerks (sleep myoclonus)
Migraine (the aura, or confusional and basilar artery variants)	benign myoclonus of infancy
Narcolepsy	benign sleep myoclonus (neonatal and infantile)

Cardiac arrhythmias
  prolonged QT syndrome
  Wolff–Parkinson–White syndrome
  supraventricular tachycardias
	benign familial paroxysmal kinesogenic choreoathetosis
	
	benign paroxysmal vertigo
	
	gastroesophageal reflux (Sandifer's syndrome)

Munchausen's syndrome by proxy (active)	cardiac arrhythmias
	non-epileptic (psychogenic or dissociative) seizures
	Munchausen's syndrome by proxy (passive)

Table 3.2 Differential diagnosis of epilepsy in adults

Syncope
  Reflex syncope
    postural
    'psychogenic'
    micturition syncope
    Valsava
  Cardiac syncope
    arrhythmias (heart block, tachycardias, etc.)
    valvular disease (especially aortic stenosis)
    cardiomyopathies
    shunts
  Perfusion failure
    hypovolemia
    syndrome of autonomic failure

Psychogenic non-epileptic seizures (PNES)
  Dissociative seizures
  Panic attacks
  Hyperventilation

Transient ischemic attacks

Migraine

Narcolepsy

Hypoglycemia

and tics/motor habits are commonly diagnosed as epilepsy (Table 3.1). Although no single feature differentiates these conditions from epilepsy, a careful account of the circumstances of the events should permit an accurate clinical diagnosis.

Differences between seizures and other paroxysmal disorders

Epileptic seizures can present in many different ways depending on the epilepsy syndrome, and the localization of focal epilepsies. The principle remains that epilepsy is a clinical diagnosis, and can be differentiated from other common paroxysmal disorders in the majority of cases without investigations.

There are some key features that should make the clinician suspicious that such events may be seizures, even if the events themselves are unusual. Seizures are stereotyped events that are usually brief, often occur in clusters, and may arise from sleep. The most common symptoms of epileptic seizures that may have a reasonable differential diagnosis fall into three broad categories.

(1) Patients presenting with preserved consciousness:

  (a) symptoms of fear or anxiety;

  (b) visual symptoms.

(2) Patients presenting with of brief episodes confusion.

(3) Patients presenting with falls ± shaking.

Tables 3.3–3.6 compare features that can aid differentiation of seizures from other common disorders presenting with similar symptoms.

Non-epileptic seizures

The two most common phenomena causing misdiagnoses of epilepsy in adults are syncope or non-epileptic attacks (Table 3.6).

Patients experiencing non-epileptic attacks constitute approximately 20% of the referrals to a specialist epilepsy clinic. Historical features which should alert the physician to this diagnostic possibility are listed in Table 3.7. These patients may require admission to hospital for observation and ambulatory monitoring after stopping therapy and, when diagnosis is confirmed, referral for neuropsychological counseling. An explanation is often evident in the family dynamics. If inappropriate antiepileptic drug therapy has not already been initiated, the patient management is simpler and the potentially disastrous psychosocial consequences may be avoided.

Symptomatic seizures

Acute symptomatic seizures, or provoked seizures, are events that occur at the time of a systemic insult or in close association with a brain insult. Common examples of symptomatic seizures are those related to toxic or metabolic disturbances or drug withdrawal. They may also occur in the context of an acute stroke or head injury (concussive seizures). In children reflex anoxic seizures are relatively common, often occurring following a minor head or other injury.

Unlike epilepsy, symptomatic seizures do not have a high risk of recurrence, unless the specific insult recurs, and as such do not usually require long-term antiepileptic drug treatment. Symptomatic seizures account for up to 40% of all incident seizures and the lifetime risk of acute symptomatic seizures is as high as 5% in men and 2.5% in women.

Misdiagnosis of epilepsy

The most common disorders that may cause a misdiagnosis of epilepsy are discussed in Tables 3.3–3.6. However, the diagnosis of epilepsy is not always straightforward and misdiagnosis rates can be as high as 25% in patients referred to tertiary centers. When there is uncertainty about a potential diagnosis of epilepsy a 'wait and see' policy should always be adopted. Whilst a delay in the diagnosis of genuine epilepsy rarely causes problems, false positive diagnosis may have severe psychological and socioeconomic consequences for the individual.

One of the most common reasons for the misdiagnosis of epilepsy is inadequate history taking, and not obtaining an accurate eye-witness account of features just before, at the start, throughout, and at the end of the paroxymal event(s). Over-interpretation of minor EEG abnormalities may also lead to misdiagnosis, and it should be emphasized that EEGs should be interpreted in the clinical context.

An incorrect diagnosis of epilepsy may also lead to a failure to identify alternative causes for the paroxysmal event. Particularly important and potentially dangerous are cardiac causes, such as bradyarrhythmias or the prolonged QT syndrome. All patients with episodes of loss of consciousness of uncertain cause should have at least a routine 12-lead ECG.

CLASSIFICATION OF SEIZURES AND EPILEPSY

Epilepsy may be classified according to a number of different criteria, including severity, seizure type, etiology, anatomical localization, age at onset or EEG findings. Most of the classifications used in the past were based on one or more of these criteria and were entirely arbitrary, reflecting the limited understanding of the pathophysiology of epilepsy. In addition, these classifications have been virtually unusable in clinical practice.

At present, the most generally accepted classification of seizures (Table 3.8) classifies them according to whether their onset is focal (partial) or generalized. Partial seizures are further subdivided according to whether consciousness is retained throughout the seizure (simple partial) or impaired at some point (complex partial). Partial seizures are characterized by a warning, which has some localizing value, but any partial seizure can be secondarily generalized. In contrast, primarily generalized seizures occur with no warning.

In 2001 a change to the current International League Against Epilepsy (ILAE) classifications was proposed for people with epileptic seizures and

Table 3.3 Differences between temporal lobe seizures and hyperventilation/panic attacks in a patient presenting with episodes of fear/anxiety

Feature	Hyperventilation/panic	Temporal lobe seizure
Age of onset	late childhood or later	any age
Duration	may be prolonged	usually < 3 min
Precipitating factors	stressful situations	none
Frequency	can be very frequent	tendency to cluster
Associated symptoms (e.g. sweating, parasthesia of peripheries and face, palpitations)	common	may occur
Autonomic symptoms	not usual	usual
Stereotyped symptoms	very rare	may occur
Arising from sleep	unusual	common
Associated loss of awareness/amnesia for event	do not occur	common
Associated limb or orofacial automatisms	do not occur	common

Table 3.4 Differences between occipital lobe seizures and migraine with visual aura in a patient presenting with visual symptoms. Modified with permission from reference 1

Feature	Migraine with visual aura	Occipital lobe seizure*
Prodromal symptoms	common	may occur
Duration	usually 15–60 min	often < 1 min
Very frequent (daily)	rare	can occur
Mainly colored circular patterns	rare	as a rule
Mainly black and white linear patterns	as a rule	rare
Moving to the opposite side of the visual field	none	exclusive
Expanding from the center to the periphery of a visual hemifield	as a rule	rare
Evolving to blindness	as a rule in basilar migraine	rare
Evolving to tonic deviation of eyes	none	exclusive
Evolving to impaired consciousness	rare	frequent
Associated with postictal headache	as a rule	frequent
Blindness and hemianopia without other preceding or subsequent symptoms	none	frequent
Postictal vomiting	frequent	uncommon

*Refers predominantly to late-onset occipital lobe epilepsy

Table 3.5 Differences between complex partial seizures and transient ischemic attacks with dysphasia in a patient presenting with episodes of brief confusion

Feature	Transient ischemic attack	Complex partial seizure
Age of onset	usually middle age to elderly	any
Associated vascular risk factors	common	may be present
Duration	mostly 5–30 min	usually < 1 min
Frequency	infrequent	can be very frequent
Associated loss of awareness	rare	common
Evolve to loss of consciousness	very rare	common
Associated limb or orofacial automatisms	do not occur	common
Speech impairment	during attack only	often persists following attack
Postictal confusion	generally not	common
Recovery	rapid	may be slow

epilepsy. This remains as 'work in progress' and under regular review – and, has not yet replaced the ILAE 1981 and 1989 classifications.

(1) Epileptic seizures and epilepsy syndromes are to be described and categorized according to a system that uses standardized terminology, and that is sufficiently flexible to take into account the following practical and dynamic aspects of epilepsy diagnosis:

    (a) Some patients cannot be given a recognized syndromic diagnosis.

    (b) Seizure types and syndromes change as new information is obtained.

    (c) Complete and detailed descriptions of ictal phenomenology are not always necessary.

    (d) Multiple classification schemes can, and should, be designed for specific purposes (e.g. communication and teaching, therapeutic trials, epidemiologic investigations, selection of surgical candidates, basic research, genetic characterizations).

(2) This diagnostic scheme is divided into five parts, or axes, organized to facilitate a logical clinical approach to the development of hypotheses necessary to determine the diagnostic studies and therapeutic strategies to be undertaken in individual patients:

Axis 1   Ictal phenomenology, from the Glossary of Descriptive Ictal Terminology, can be used to describe ictal events with any degree of detail needed.

Axis 2   Seizure type, from the List of Epileptic Seizures. Localization within the brain and precipitating stimuli for reflex seizures should be specified when appropriate.

Axis 3   Syndrome, from the List of Epilepsy Syndromes, with the understanding that a syndromic diagnosis may not always be possible.

Axis 4   Etiology, from a Classification of Diseases Frequently Associated with Epileptic Seizures or Epilepsy Syndromes when possible, genetic defects, or specific pathological substrates for symptomatic focal epilepsies.

Axis 5   Impairment, this is optional, but often useful, an additional diagnostic parameter can be derived from an impairment classification adapted from the WHO International Classification of Impairments, Disability and Handicaps (ICIDH)-2.

The first axis ('seizure description') will replace the terms 'simple partial' and 'complex partial' with

Table 3.6 Differences between tonic-clonic seizures, syncope and non-epileptic attacks in a patient presenting with falls ± shaking

Feature	Syncope	Psychogenic non-epileptic seizures (PNES)	Tonic-clonic seizure
Posture	upright (usually)	any	any
Pallor and sweating	invariable	may occur	may occur
Onset	gradual	may be gradual	sudden/aura
Injury	rare	uncommon	not uncommon
Lateral tongue biting	rare	rare	not uncommon
Limb or body jerks	common (but few)	common	common
Retained consciousness in prolonged event	not usually prolonged	common	very rare
Other movements* (e.g. pelvic thrusting, asynchronous thrashing limb movements, rolling movements)	rare	common	rare
Movements waxing and waning	rare	common	rare
Cyanosis	rare	rare	common
Stereotypical attacks	can occur	may occur	usual
Incontinence	can occur	can occur	common
Unconsciousness†	seconds	often many minutes	minutes
Gaze aversion	rare	common	rare
Resistance to passive limb movement or eye-opening	rare	common	unusual
Prevention of hand falling on face	rare	common	unusual
Induced by suggestion	unusual	common	rare
Recovery	rapid	may be prolonged	often slow
Postictal confusion	rare	may be absent	common
Frequency	infrequent	frequent	may be frequent
Ictal EEG abnormality	none	none	typically
Postictal EEG abnormality	rarely	rarely	common
Precipitating factors	crowded places, lack of food, unpleasant circumstances	stress, sexual abuse	rare

*Brief myoclonic or clonic movements occur in 80% of patients with syncope. Unlike an epileptic convulsion, however, recovery is rapid; †Occasionally, syncope may result in a more prolonged period of cerebral hypoxia, which may cause an anoxic tonic-clonic seizure with a longer duration of unconsciousness and a slower rate of recovery

'focal' and the precise semiology of the seizure will then be described in detail. This will include specifically whether consciousness is fully preserved, impaired or lost during the focal seizure. This pro- posed revised classification also includes several additional seizure types and epilepsy syndromes that were not included in the earlier, 1981 and 1989 classification.

Table 3.7 Factors associated with psychogenic non-epileptic seizures (also called dissociative seizures)

Attacks
Adult onset
Variable*
Bizarre eye-witness descriptions
Circumstantial (provoked by stress)
Dramatic events
Recurrent hospitalization
No response or worse on antiepileptic drugs

Patient/past medical history
Female gender
Paramedical occupation
Traumatic childhood
Major life stressors (divorce, bereavement)
Past history of unexplained physical symptoms
Past psychiatric history, especially of self-abuse

Examination/investigation
Normal neurological examination
Evidence of illness behavior
EEG normal or non-specifically abnormal
CT scan normal

---

*Whilst commonly the nature of non-epileptic attacks varies considerably there may be a degree of stereotypy amongst individual patients, for example, 'flailers', 'tremblers', 'swooners'

Table 3.8 Classification of seizures. With permission from reference 2

Partial seizures (beginning locally)
Simple (consciousness unimpaired)
  with motor symptoms
  with somatosensory or special sensory symptoms
  with autonomic symptoms
  with psychic symptoms
Complex (consciousness impaired)
  beginning as simple partial seizures, but progressing to complex seizures
  with impaired consciousness at onset
    impairment of consciousness only
    with automatisms
Partial but becoming secondarily generalized

Generalized seizures
Absence
  typical ('petit mal')
  atypical
Myoclonic
Clonic
Tonic
Tonic-clonic
Atonic

EPILEPSY SYNDROMES

The concept of epilepsy syndromes was first considered in 1985. In 1989, the ILAE revised the classification of epilepsy by incorporating epilepsy syndromes in an attempt to simplify classification (Table 3.9). The syndromic approach is retained in the 2001 proposed revised classification but with some changes.

A syndrome is a cluster of signs and symptoms that non-fortuitously occur together. An epileptic syndrome is characterized by both clinical and EEG findings.

(1) Clinical findings

　(a)　Seizure type(s);

　(b)　Age at onset;

　(c)　Neurological findings;

　(d)　Family history.

(2) EEG findings include:

　(a)　Interictal;

　(b)　Ictal.

Delineation of the epilepsy syndromes permits a greater precision of diagnosis and, more importantly, of prognosis than does the simple classification of seizure types. The same type of seizure can occur in different syndromes, but different types of seizure can also belong to the same syndrome.

The concept of epilepsy syndromes is fundamentally pragmatic and helps in selecting the appropriate investigations, deciding on the optimal antiepileptic treatment and predicting the outcome. The concept of syndromes also has value in dispensing with the other parameters or assumptions regarding the pathogenesis of epilepsy. Finally, the use of epilepsy syndromes is useful in research and comparative studies.

However, there are a number of potential deficiencies in the application of epilepsy syndromes. First, epilepsy syndromes do not provide any information as to the underlying etiology. West's syndrome, for example, may be caused by at least 30

Table 3.9 International League Against Epilepsy revised classification of epilepsy. With permission from reference 3

---

(1) *Localization-related (focal, local, partial) epilepsies and syndromes*

    1.1   Idiopathic (with age-related onset)

           benign childhood epilepsy with centrotemporal spikes

           childhood epilepsy with occipital paroxysms

           primary reading epilepsy

    1.2   Symptomatic

           chronic progressive epilepsia partialis continua of childhood (Koshevnikoff's syndrome)

           syndromes characterized by seizures with specific modes of presentation

    1.3   Cryptogenic (presumed symptomatic but etiology unknown)

(2) *Generalized epilepsies and syndromes*

    2.1   Idiopathic (with age-related onset, listed in order of age)

           benign neonatal familial convulsions

           benign neonatal convulsions

           benign myoclonic epilepsy in infancy

           childhood absence epilepsy

           juvenile absence epilepsy

           juvenile myoclonic epilepsy

           epilepsy with grand mal (generalized tonic-clonic) seizures on awakening

           other generalized idiopathic epilepsies not defined above

           epilepsies with seizures precipitated by specific modes of activation (reflex and reading epilepsies)

    2.2   Cryptogenic or symptomatic (in order of age)

           West's syndrome

           Lennox–Gastaut syndrome

           epilepsy with myoclonic-astatic seizures

           epilepsy with myoclonic absences

    2.3   Symptomatic

        2.3.1   Non-specific etiology

              early myoclonic encephalopathy

              early infantile epileptic encephalopathy with suppression burst

              other symptomatic generalized epilepsies not defined above

        2.3.2   Specific syndromes/etiologies

              cerebral malformations

              inborn errors of metabolism including pyridoxine dependency, glucose transport protein and biotinidase deficiencies and disorders frequently presenting as progressive myoclonic epilepsy

continued

different conditions. Second, adherence to the criteria of any specific syndrome is essential; forcing an atypical case into a generally accepted syndrome is to be avoided as this will defeat the process and also the objective of delineating and defining a 'real' and identifiable epilepsy syndrome.

Some syndromes have common signs and a predictable outcome, for example, West's syndrome and Lennox–Gastaut syndrome, benign rolandic epilepsy, late-onset benign occipital epilepsy and severe myoclonic epilepsy of infancy. Others, such as absence seizures, are less specific and may include several subgroups with different outcomes and different associated features. Still others are, in fact, only loose collections of a few common characteristics inconsistently linked to one another.

The emphasis placed on epilepsy syndromes is justified by the inadequacies and difficulties of the traditional approach to epilepsy, which is based on seizure types and the search for an underlying lesion. However, if the concept of epilepsy syndromes is to be of any practical use, it has to be limited to those

Table 3.9 *Continued*

(3) *Epilepsies and syndromes undetermined as to whether focal or generalized*
    3.1   With both generalized and focal seizures
        neonatal seizures
        severe myoclonic epilepsy in infancy (Figure 3.1)
        epilepsy with continuous spike waves during slow-wave sleep (Figure 3.2)
        acquired epileptic aphasia (Landau–Kleffner syndrome)
        other undetermined epilepsies not defined above
    3.2   Without unequivocal generalized or focal features

(4) *Special syndromes*
    4.1   Situation-related seizures
        febrile convulsions
        isolated seizures or isolated status epilepticus
        seizures occurring only when there is an acute metabolic or toxic event due to factors such as alcohol, drugs,
          eclampsia, non-ketotic hyperglycemia
        reflex epilepsy

electroclinical clusters that are unequivocally identifiable.

With the current advances in DNA and genetic studies, the idea of epilepsy syndromes may eventually become redundant to be replaced by specific epileptic disorders. However, for the present, they serve to simplify the classification of epilepsy and are of pragmatic value.

Classification of syndromes

Syndromic classification divides the epilepsies into two broad categories: localization-related and generalized. Each category is further subdivided into idiopathic, symptomatic and cryptogenic. Idiopathic epilepsies are age-related and have well-defined EEG characteristics, whereas symptomatic/cryptogenic epilepsies occur at any age and have no typical EEG features. Four broad categories of epilepsy syndrome are described.

Idiopathic generalized epilepsies commence in the first, second and third decades of life. Affected subjects usually have no associated intellectual or neurological deficits. These syndromes have a favorable prognosis with most patients responding to sodium valproate or lamotrigine. The genetic bases of these syndromes have been well established and, although there is some overlap, twin studies indicate that specific syndromes are inherited within families.

Symptomatic generalized epilepsies are age-dependent encephalopathies characterized by onset in infancy/early childhood, and poor prognoses for both seizure control and development. Although these are distinct electroclinical entities, there is a degree of overlap. It is possible that these represent different responses to a wide range of insults at different stages of cerebral maturation.

Idiopathic partial epilepsies commence in childhood and include both the very commonly seen benign epilepsy of childhood with centrotemporal spikes and the slightly less common childhood epilepsy with occipital paroxysms. Both carry particularly benign prognoses.

Symptomatic partial epilepsies occur at any age with the most likely cause determined by the age of onset. Approximately 30% of cases of childhood epilepsy fall into this category. Adult-onset partial epilepsy is assumed to be symptomatic, although the cause often remains elusive.

Syndromic classification is less useful in these epilepsies where the most important consideration is definition of the cause which, in turn, determines the prognosis and influences management.

Adult-onset idiopathic generalized epilepsy (JGE). characteristically presents in the first two decades of life. Rarely, this may occur as late as the fifth decade and some studies have reported up to 30% of patients with IGE having their first seizure at over 20 years of age. Absence seizures are difficult to recognize in adults as they are often so brief and clinically insignificant. If they are apparent, they will

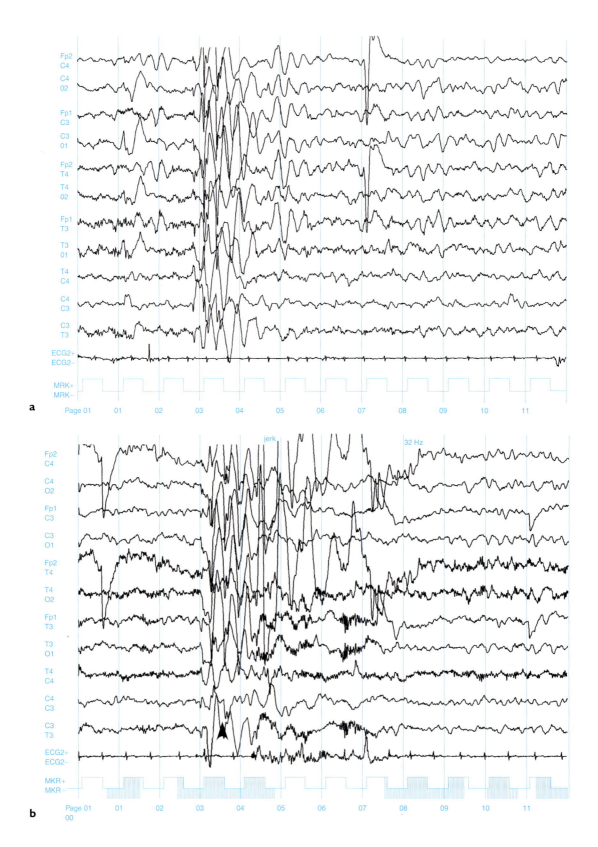

Figure 3.1 EEG of a 16-month-old infant with probable severe myoclonic epilepsy in infancy. The patient had two generalized and prolonged febrile seizures at 6 and 7 months of age, and then presented at 13 months of age with weekly partial, secondarily generalized tonic-clonic and myoclonic seizures. An EEG was normal at 13 months of age. The EEG at 16 months of age showed a diffusely slow background and frequent, high amplitude, generalized spike and slow-wave discharges (a) and possible photosensitivity with a myoclonic seizure affecting the patient's trunk (b) (arrow)

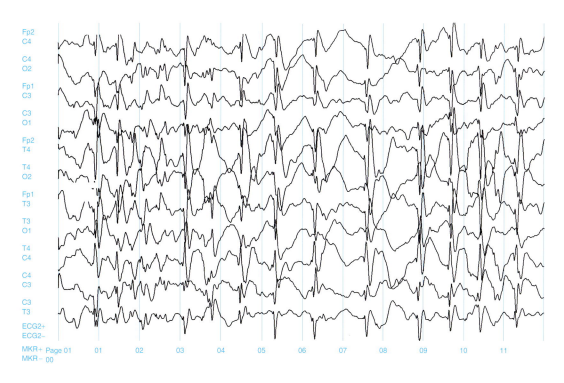

Figure 3.2 Sleeping EEG of a 10-year-old boy with an 18-month history of infrequent nocturnal, focal seizures and a 6-month history of regression in both receptive and expressive language skills showing electrical status epilepticus of slow-wave sleep (ESESS). The patient was not being treated with an antiepileptic drug at the time of this EEG. An earlier EEG undertaken after his third focal seizure had been reported as being 'consistent with benign partial epilepsy with centro-temporal spikes'

often be misinterpreted as complex partial seizures in this age group. Otherwise, the clinical syndromes are similar to those with a younger age of onset and also seem to have a similarly good prognosis.

Examples of the commonly encountered age-related epilepsy syndromes are shown in Figures 3.3–3.21.

The current classification of the epilepsy syndromes may also be revised in the future based on work in progress arising out of the proposal of the ILAE Task Force on Classification and Terminology[6]. A specific change recommended by the ILAE Task Force is to replace the term 'cryptogenic' with 'probably symptomatic'. Therefore the epilepsy syndromes or epilepsies can be classified in terms of 'idiopathic', 'symptomatic' or 'probably symptomatic'.

DETERMINATION OF CAUSE

Epilepsy is a symptom not a diagnosis *per se*. An underlying cause must always be considered,

although one will not always be found. An etiological classification of seizures and epilepsy is shown in Table 3.10.

Many cerebral pathologies may cause acute symptomatic seizures and, subsequently, epilepsy (Table 3.11). Acute symptomatic seizures may occur in response to a number of systemic disturbances (Table 3.12).

Unselected population-based studies indicate that the cause can be identified in approximately one-third of cases. The etiology may be inferred from

Table 3.10 Classification of seizures and epilepsy by etiology

Acute symptomatic seizures
Isolated cryptogenic seizures
Epilepsies
remote symptomatic
genetic
cryptogenic

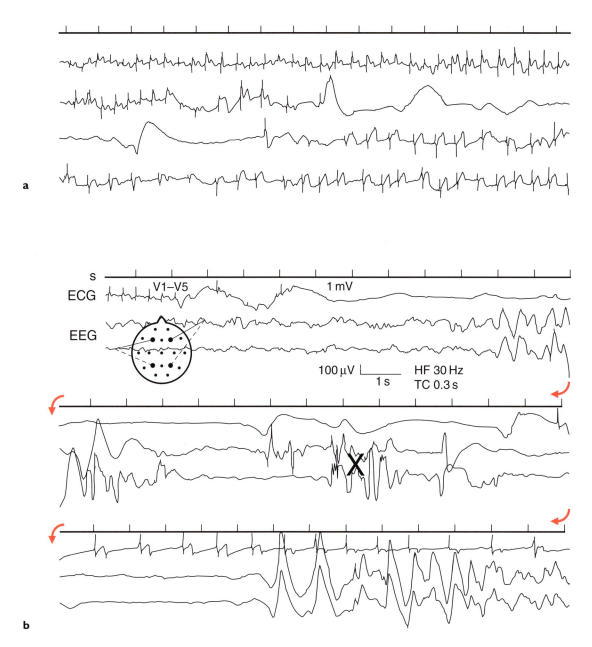

Figure 3.3 Continuous ambulatory ECG (a) of a 2-year-old boy, whose frequent episodes of loss of consciousness with rigidity began at age 9 months, taken during a seizure induced by a head bump; such an association with head bumps or other painful stimuli was not recognized for many months. From top to bottom: a time marker (s); consecutive 16-s epochs; 14 s asystole preceded by 3 s of relative bradycardia. The simultaneous EEG (not shown) showed 6–7 s of electrical silence. Cassette EEG/ECG (b) of a tonic seizure induced by a head bump. Onset of asystole is preceded by 2 s of relative brady-cardia and followed by, after 20 s of standstill, a nodal escape rhythm. EEG flattening lasts for 18 s before the abrupt return of cerebral activity 6 s after restoration of ECG. There is no 'epileptic' spiking. Modified with permission from reference 4

the clinical history, which should include direct questioning on perinatal history and development, complex early febrile convulsions (prolonged, focal or multiple episodes within 24 h)[7], previous severe head injury, central nervous system infection, family history of epilepsy and the recent development of other neurological symptoms and signs.

Age of onset is the most important indicator both of the likelihood of epilepsy being symptomatic and of the probable cause (Figure 3.21).

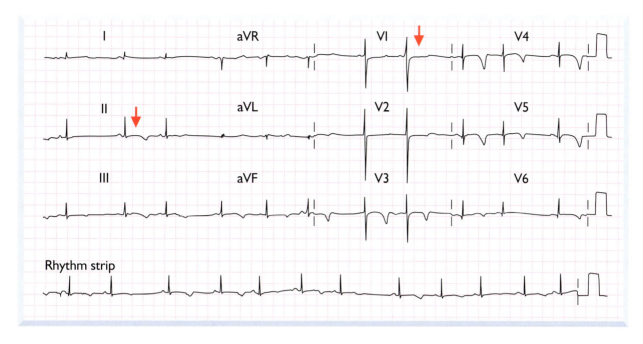

Figure 3.4 ECG of an 11-year-old boy who had frequent episodes of blackouts or 'faints', particularly during athletics and just after swimming. There is prolongation of the QT interval (arrowed). A similar appearance was seen in his father's ECG. The diagnosis was Romano–Ward syndrome (congenital prolongation of the QT interval)

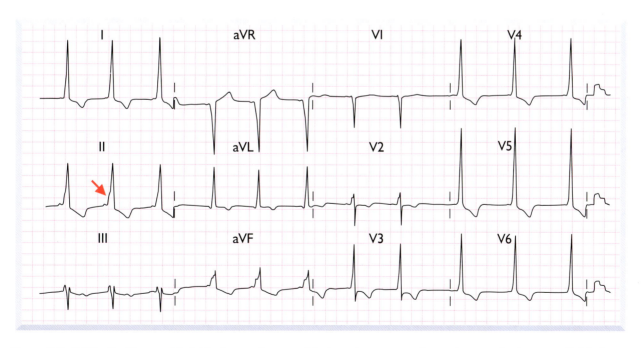

Figure 3.5 ECG of a 12-year-old child whose infrequent 'blackouts' were treated as epilepsy with phenytoin. ECG shows Wolff–Parkinson–White syndrome with a short PR interval and delta wave (arrow)

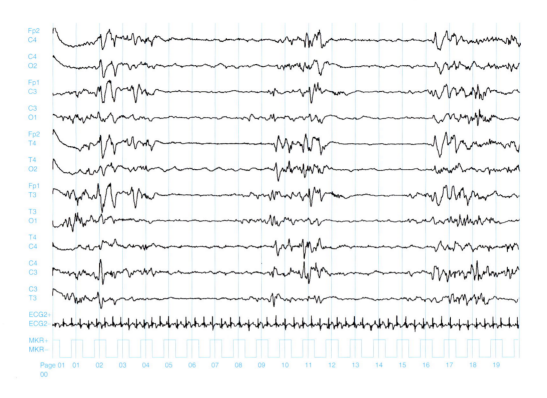

Figure 3.6 EEG of a 6-week-old infant with intrauterine growth retardation born at 37 weeks' gestation and who developed a moderately severe hypoxic–ischemic encephalopathy (HIE) and multiple organ dysfunction followed by drug-resistant seizures and profound irritability. Waking EEG demonstrates a burst-suppression pattern (the periods of 'suppression' are briefer than usual in children with HIE). No clinical seizures occurred during the 'bursts'

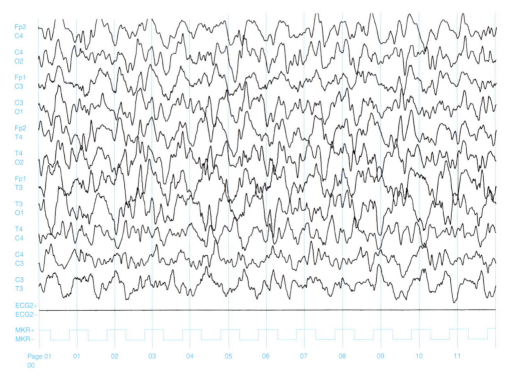

Figure 3.7 EEG of an 8-month-old boy with infantile spasms and developmental delay (West's syndrome) due to tuberous sclerosis. There is hypsarrhythmia (chaotic disorganized background, multifocal high-amplitude spikes and slow waves)

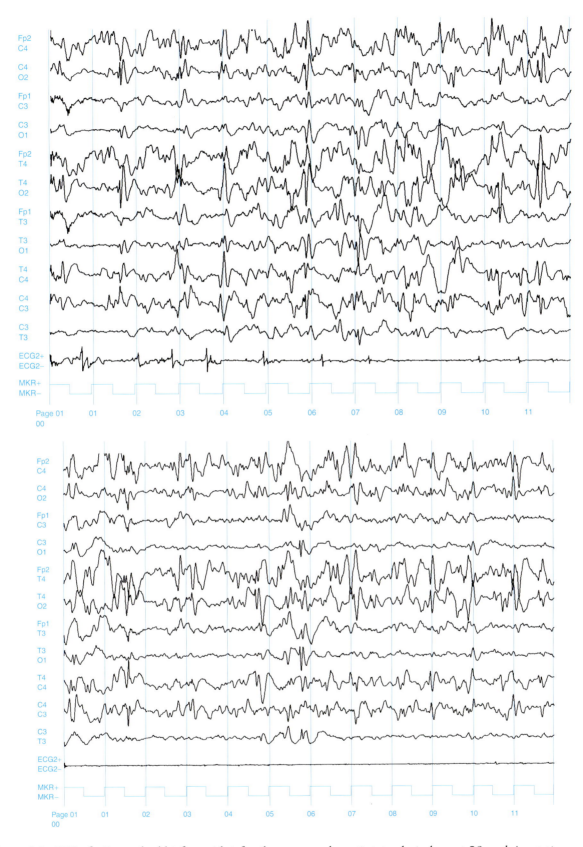

Figure 3.8 EEG of a 7-month-old infant with infantile spasms and spastic tetraplegia, born at 26 weeks' gestation complicated by bilateral intraventricular hemorrhages and a large right temporoparietal intraparenchymal hemorrhage. EEG demonstrates bilateral abnormalities but unilateral (right) hypsarrhythmia, consistent with 'atypical' or 'modified' hypsarrhythmia

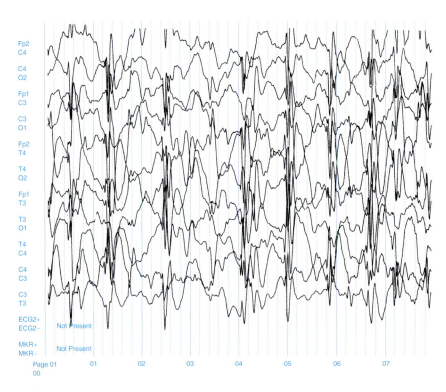

Figure 3.9 EEG of a 10-month-old infant with cryptogenic infantile spasms (unknown etiology) demonstrating atypical hypsarrhythmia with a subtle 'burst-suppression' pattern. Non-ketotic hyperglycinemia was excluded with a normal CSF : blood glycine ratio and normal liver biopsy. Spasm control was never achieved

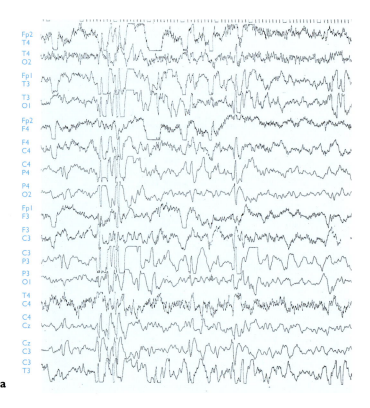

Figure 3.10 EEGs of a 3-year-old girl with myoclonic-astatic epilepsy showing generalized spike and slow-wave activity, and polyspike discharge accompanied by slight head-drop and bilateral 'jerks' of the legs (a) *continued*

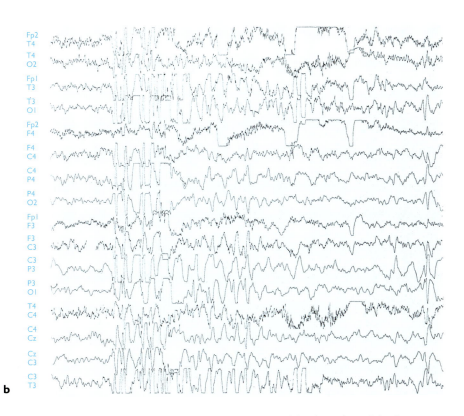

Figure 3.10 *Continued* a further similar discharge is accompanied by a jerk backwards with both arms outstretched (b)

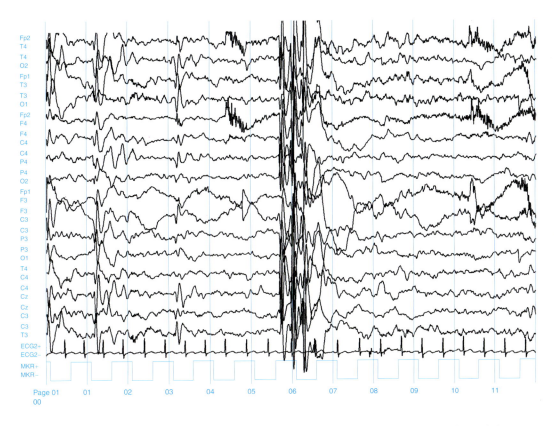

Figure 3.11 EEG of a 7-year-old girl with myoclonic astatic epilepsy showing generalized spike and slow wave and also polyspike and slow-wave activity without any clinical seizure

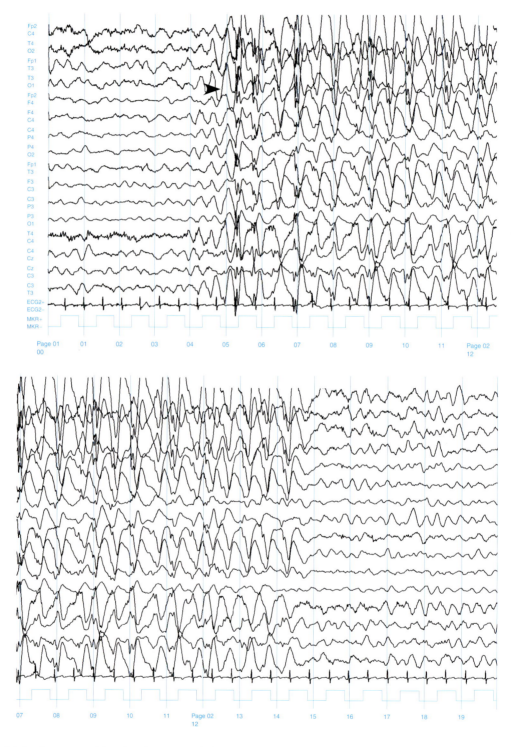

Figure 3.12 EEG of a 9-year-old girl with a 9-month history of drug-resistant tonic-clonic, absence and infrequent atonic seizures showing an electroclinical episode characterized by a generalized (bi-frontal) onset of slow, spike and slow-wave activity at 1.5–2 Hz on a diffusely slow background for the child's age. At the onset (arrow), the patient stopped talking, her head fell forward slightly and she showed very subtle myoclonus affecting her face and head that persisted throughout the 10-s episode; it has not been possible definitively to identify an epilepsy syndrome (?myoclonic astatic epilepsy)

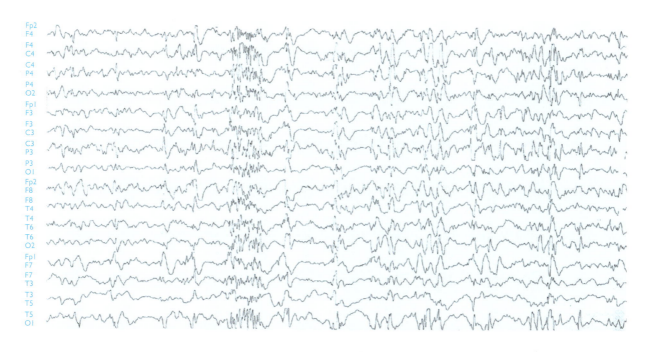

Figure 3.13 Sleeping EEG of a 6-year-old boy with Lennox–Gastaut syndrome (tonic, atonic, myoclonic and generalized tonic-clonic seizures, and severe learning difficulties) shows multiple discharges of polyspike and spike–wave complexes

Table 3.11 Central nervous system disease causing seizures and epilepsy. With permission from reference 5

Congenital	hypoxic-ischemic cerebral insult
	birth trauma, tuberous sclerosis
	arteriovenous malformation
	lipid-storage diseases
	leukodystrophies
	Down syndrome
Infective	meningitis, encephalitis
	abscess, syphilis
Trauma	diffuse brain injury, hematoma (extradural,
	subdural, intracerebral)
	depressed skull fracture
Tumor	glioma, meningioma
	secondary carcinoma, etc.
Vascular	atheroma, arteritis, aneurysm
Degenerative	Alzheimer's, Batten's, Creutzfeldt–Jakob,
	Pick's diseases, etc.
Miscellaneous	demyelination

Table 3.12 Systemic disturbances causing seizures

Fever	Drugs
Hypoxia	Drug withdrawal
Hypoglycemia	Toxins
Electrolyte imbalance	
	Pyridoxine deficiency
Renal failure	Porphyria
Hepatic failure	Inborn errors of metabolism
Respiratory failure	

The principal role of EEG in epilepsy is in the classification of seizures/epilepsy. However, the presence of a focal slow- or spike-wave abnormality should raise the suspicion of a structural lesion and suggests the need for imaging, although there is a low correlation between a focal sharp wave or spike and identifying a structural lesion, particularly in children. There is a higher correlation between a focal slow-wave discharge (particularly if rhythmic) and a space-occupying lesion such as a tumor.

There is no place for a policy of unselected computed tomography (CT) or magnetic resonance

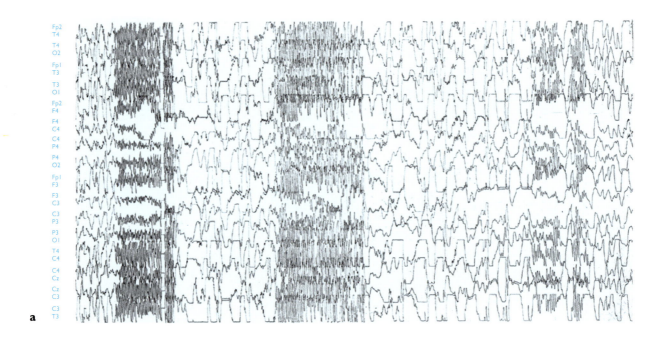

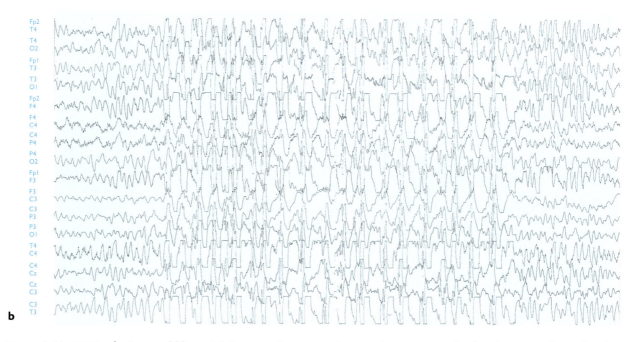

Figure 3.14 EEGs of a 9-year-old boy with Lennox–Gastaut syndrome, who experienced infantile spasms during his first year of life, show irregular diffuse spike and slow-wave activity (b). This was accompanied by an episode of atypical absence (unresponsive, with twitching of eyelids, chin and fingers) and a burst of rapid rhythm (10 cps) accompanied by a brief 'salaam'-type seizure or epileptic spasm (a)

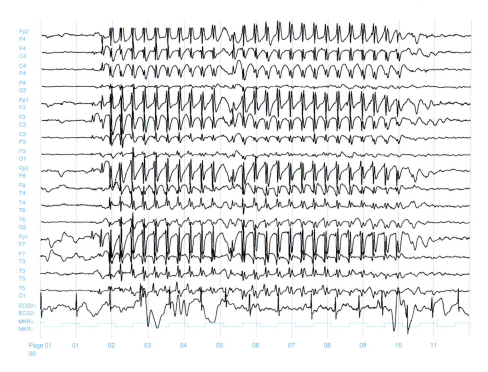

Figure 3.15 EEG of a 7-year-old girl with childhood-onset absence epilepsy (CAE) showing generalized, rhythmic spike and slow-wave activity at a frequency of 3 Hz. The appearance of a possible left frontal onset at Fp1-F3 is often seen in patients with a primary generalized epilepsy. The patient was unresponsive during the episode and demonstrated some automatisms (licking her lips). Seizure control has been difficult. This should be contrasted with the EEG of another patient with childhood-onset absence epilepsy (Figure 3.16) where there is a bi-occipital onset to the generalized spike and slow-wave activity

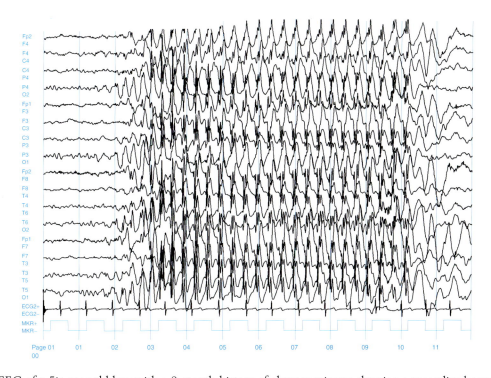

Figure 3.16 EEG of a 5½-year-old boy with a 9-month history of absence seizures showing a generalized onset of rhythmic spike and slow-wave activity with a frequency of 3 Hz; the onset appears to be bi-occipital rather than frontal as seen in the patient whose EEG is shown in Figure 3.15. This patient's absences have been easily controlled with lamotrigine monotherapy

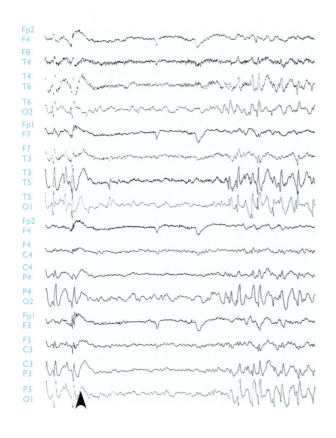

Figure 3.17 EEG of an 8-year-old girl who had a 4-month history of nocturnal partial seizures characterized by eye deviation, hemiconvulsions and secondary generalization (tonic-clonic convulsions). She also experienced seizures during the day which began with a visual 'aura' (fortification spectra or 'colored lights') and were followed, within 1–2 min, by brief clonic movements (unilateral or bilateral) and a severe headache. Generalized tonic-clonic seizures occasionally followed the initial visual aura. Although migraine was initially diagnosed, the patient in fact has benign childhood epilepsy with occipital paroxysms (late-onset occipital epilepsy), comprising high-amplitude runs of repetitive irregular occipital spikes or sharp- and slow-wave complexes occurring bilaterally and tending to attenuate on eye opening (arrowed)

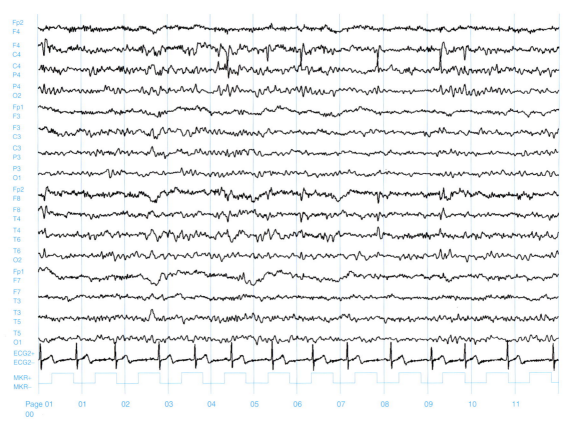

Figure 3.18 EEG of an 8-year-old boy with a 6-month history consistent with benign partial epilepsy with centrotemporal (rolandic) spikes showing a frequent right frontotemporal/posterior frontal sharp wave or spike discharge

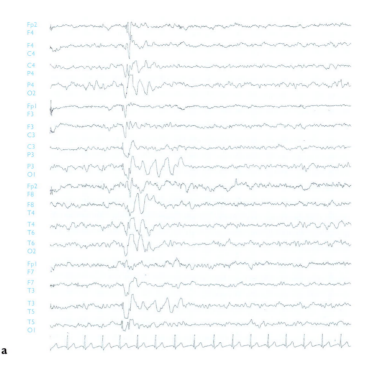

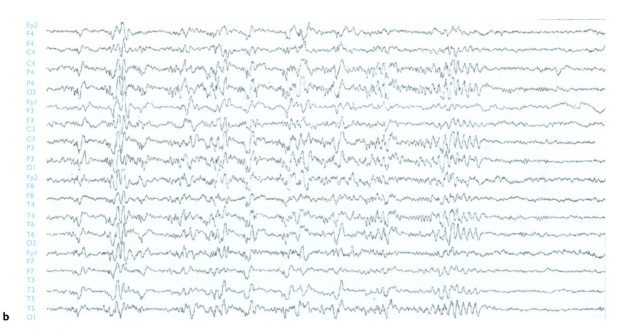

Figure 3.19 EEGs of a 12-year-old boy with juvenile myoclonic epilepsy showing an irregular spike–wave complex during rest (a), and photosensitivity (unaccompanied by any clinical change) during photic stimulation (b)

imaging (MRI) scanning in patients with epilepsy as clinically relevant abnormalities are rarely detected by this technology. However, CT – or, preferably, MRI – is indicated in patients with later-onset partial seizures with or without neurological signs or focal EEG abnormalities, particularly in those who do not respond to treatment.

Magnetic resonance imaging (MRI) is far superior to CT in the detection of small structural and subtle atrophic lesions, but is generally inferior to CT in demonstrating intracerebral calcification and acute hemorrhage. MRI is an essential part of presurgical investigation protocols, and is the imaging modality of choice when undertaking structural radiological

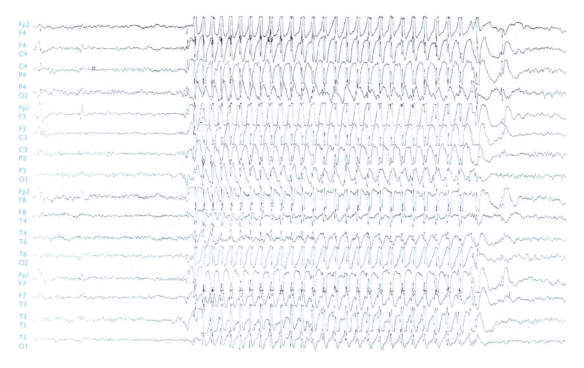

Figure 3.20 EEG of a 13-year-old girl who had a 6-month history of 'blanks', and two generalized tonic-clonic seizures within a couple of hours of waking (juvenile-onset absence epilepsy). There is a generalized discharge of spike and slow-wave activity at 3 cps, accompanied by eye-opening, lip-smacking and a sigh

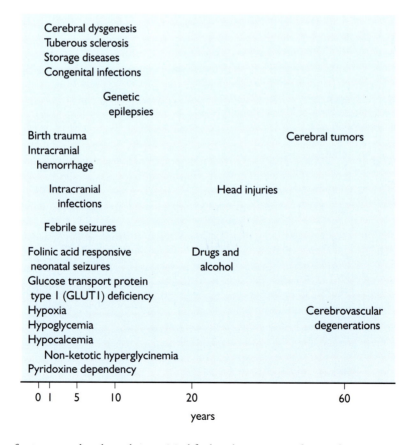

Figure 3.21 Causes of seizures and epilepsy by age. Modified with permission from reference 5

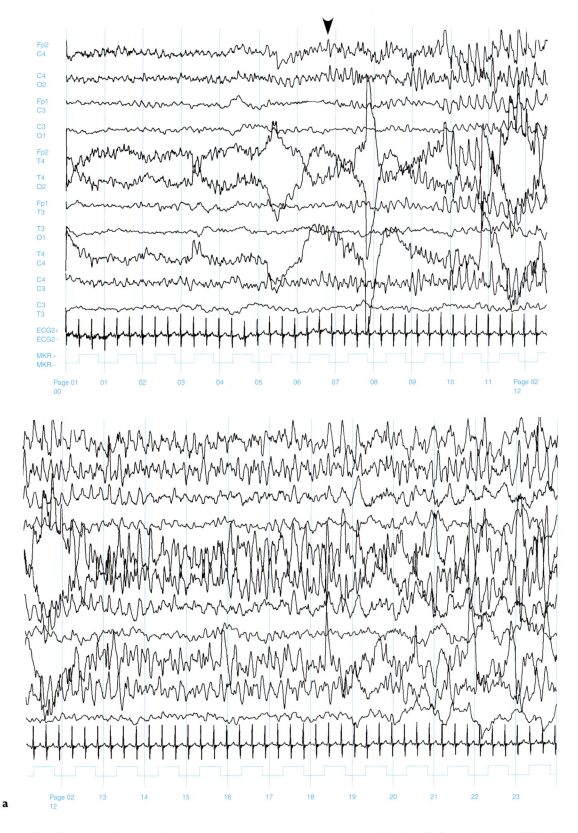

Figure 3.22 EEG of an 18-week-old infant with migrating partial seizures (epilepsy) of infancy that recorded both a right (a) frontotemporal partial seizure (arrow) and a much briefer left (b) temporal partial seizure (arrow). Seizure onset had been from 5 weeks of age. The frequency ranged from 10 to over 60 partial seizures every day and the seizures were resistant to all antiepileptic drugs (including high dose prednisolone, intravenous immunoglobulins, pyridoxal phosphate) and the 'classical' ketogenic diet *(Continued)*

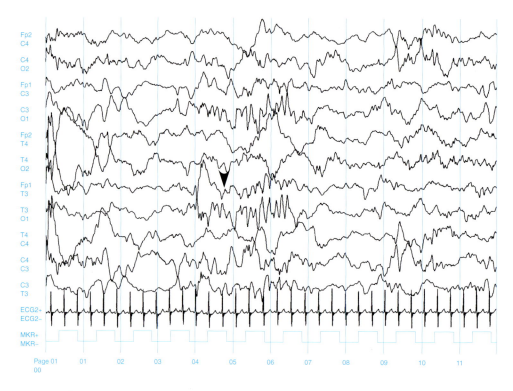

Figure 3.22 *Continued*

investigation of patients (of all ages) with epilepsy. An independent role for functional imaging (single-photon emission computed tomography (SPECT) and positron emission tomography (PET)) remains undefined and these imaging modalities may well be replaced by functional MRI (fMRI) over the next decade.

Unfortunately, there remain a number of adults and children with epilepsy and specific epilepsy syndromes, where no cause is identified despite exhaustive radiological, biochemical and genetic investigations; a specific example is migrating partial seizures (epilepsy) of infancy (Figure 3.22).

REFERENCES

1. Panayiotopoulos CP. Visual phenomena and headache in occipital epilepsy: a review, a systematic study and differentiation from migraine. Epileptic Disord 1999; 1: 205–16

2. Commission on Classification and Terminology of the International League Against Epilepsy. Proposal for revised clinical and electroencephalographic classification of epilepsy seizures. Epilepsia 1981; 22: 489–501

3. Commission on classification and Terminology of the International League Against Epilepsy. Proposal for classification of epilepsies and epileptic syndromes. Epilepsia 1989; 30: 389–99

4. Stephenson JBP. Fits and Faints. London: MacKeith Press, 1990: 103

5. Chadwick D. Paroxysmal disorders. In Chadwick D, Cartlidge NEF, Bates D, eds. Medical Neurology. Edinburgh: Churchill Livingstone, 1989: 152–85

6. Engel J Jr. A proposed diagnostic scheme for people with epileptic seizures and with epilepsy: report of the ILAE Task Force on Classification and Terminology. Epilepsia 2001; 42: 796–803

7. Waruiru C, Appleton R. Febrile seizures – an update. Arch Dis Child 2004; 89: 751–6

FURTHER READING

1. Roger J, Bureau M, Dravet C, et al. Epileptic Syndromes in Infancy, Childhood and Adolescence, 3rd edn. Eastleigh, UK: John Libbey, 2002

2. Panayiotopoulos CP. The epilepsies: seizures, syndromes and management based on the ILAE classifications and practice parameter guidelines. Oxfordshire: Bladon Medical Publishing, 2005

4. Etiology

INTRODUCTION

Epilepsy is a symptom, not a diagnosis, and not caused by a single disorder. Epilepsy may be due to virtually any cerebral pathology, and seizures may occur in association with a large number of systemic disorders. Although there are many causes of recurrent seizures and epilepsy, including cerebral hypoxia at birth, central nervous system (CNS) infections, head trauma and brain tumors, no specific etiology can be found in almost two-thirds of patients.

This chapter reflects the heterogeneity of causes of epilepsy with an emphasis on clinicopathological correlations.

PERINATAL CAUSES

The newborn period is the time of life with the highest risk of seizures and epilepsy. The immature and developing brain is susceptible to a number of insults, including:

(1) *Asphyxia (hypoxic–ischemic encephalopathy)* This is the most common and also the most serious cause of neonatal seizures. Asphyxia usually occurs in term or postmature infants. The changes are those of necrosis of the deep cerebral white matter due to intrauterine or perinatal cerebral hypoxia, or ischemia. Figures 4.1–4.4 illustrate the increasing severity of damage. Infantile spasms frequently develop at between 5 and 8 months of age.

(2) *Intra- and periventricular hemorrhage* This phenomenon occurs predominantly in preterm infants (Figures 4.5–4.8).

(3) *Transient metabolic dysfunction* This may occur, for example, in hypoglycemia, hypocalcemia or hyponatremia.

(4) *Sepsis* This may arise from congenital infections such as TORCH syndrome (*Toxoplasma* (Figure 4.9), Other, Rubella, Cytomegalovirus

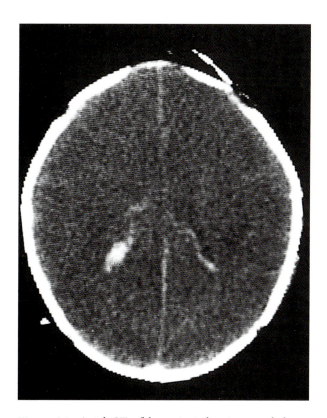

Figure 4.1 Axial CT of hypoxic–ischemic encephalopathy in a 24-h-old infant, born at week 42 of gestation following an antepartum hemorrhage. The brain is markedly swollen with no white–gray matter differentiation. Seizures developed 4 h after birth and persisted until death 3 days later

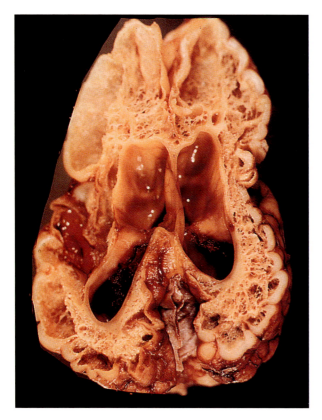

Figure 4.2 Cystic encephalomalacia. All of the cerebral white matter has been reduced to a honeycomb of cystic cavities traversed by gliovascular strands

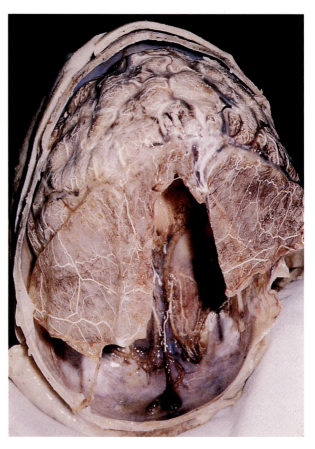

Figure 4.4 Gross appearance of the cerebrum in porencephaly removed at autopsy

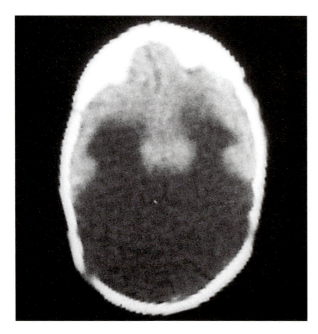

Figure 4.3 CT of porencephaly shows loss of much of the substance of the cerebrum, which has been replaced by bilateral cystic cavities covered by leptomeninges which communicate with the ventricular system

(Figures 4.10–4.12) and Herpes), and from syphilis, septicemia or meningitis.

(5) *Cerebral malformations/dysgenesis* These include hemimegalencephaly (Figures 4.13 and 4.14), lissencephaly (Figures 4.15 and 4.16), neuronal migration disorders (Figure 4.17), schizencephaly (Figures 4.18 and 4.19), Aicardi syndrome (Figure 4.20) and agenesis of the corpus callosum (Figures 4.21–4.23), hypothalamic hamartoma (Figure 4.24), holoprosencephaly (Figures 4.25–4.27) and temporal lobe agenesis (Figure 4.28). The most common malformations of cortical development to present with epilepsy will be discussed in more detail in the section on genetic epilepsies.

It is the etiology of the seizures, rather than the seizures themselves, that is the predicting factor in the determination of 'late' epilepsy and intellectual status. The risk of late epilepsy is much greater if neonatal seizures were caused by hypoxic–ischemic encephalopathy or a cerebral malformation.

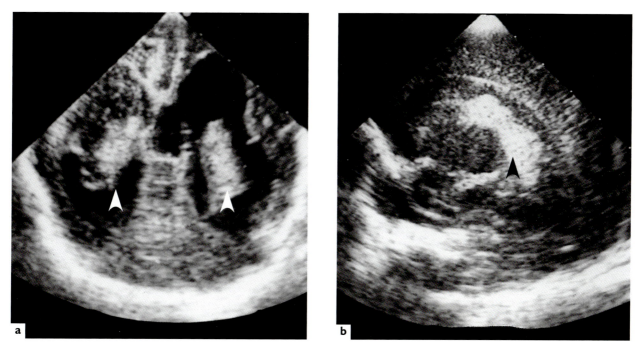

Figure 4.5 Axial (a) and parasagittal (b) cranial ultrasound scans showing ventricular dilatation and bilateral (left) intraventricular hemorrhages (arrowed) in a 6-day-old infant, born at week 28 of gestation, who presented with seizures, hypotension and sudden collapse

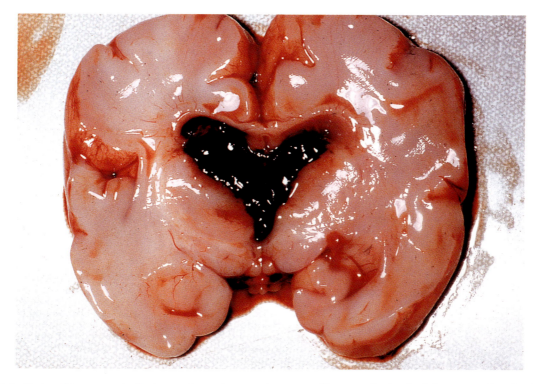

Figure 4.6 Perinatal intraventricular hemorrhage. A coronal section of brain at the level of the mammillary bodies shows the ventricles to be filled with blood. Hemorrhage into the periventricular germinal matrix and ventricles is common in perinatal hypoxic–ischemic encephalopathy

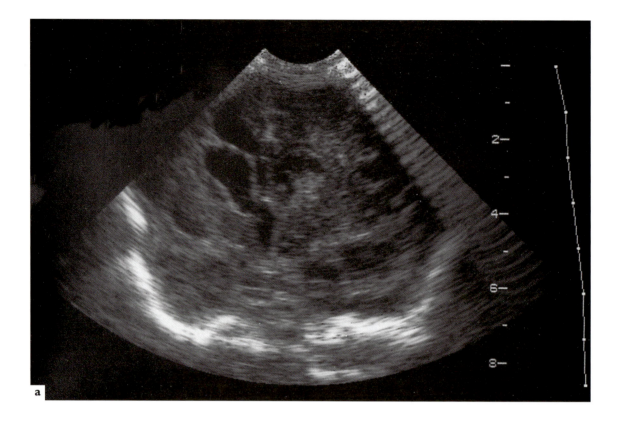

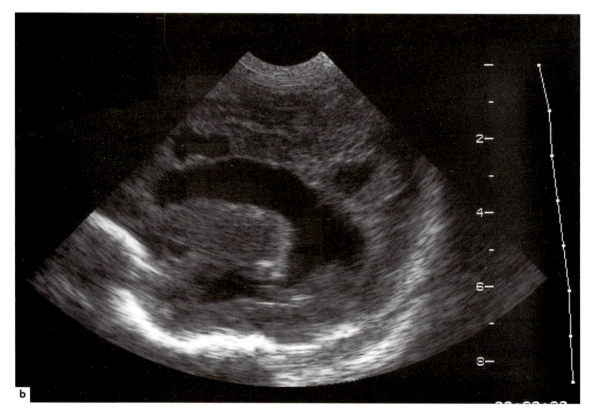

Figure 4.7 Periventricular leukomalacia. A 3-week-old boy born at week 32 of gestation presented with hypotonia, and frequent tonic and myoclonic seizures due to periventricular leukomalacia following a periventricular hemorrhage. Coronal (a) and parasagittal (b) cranial ultrasound scans show irregular and enlarged lateral ventricles and numerous cystic spaces

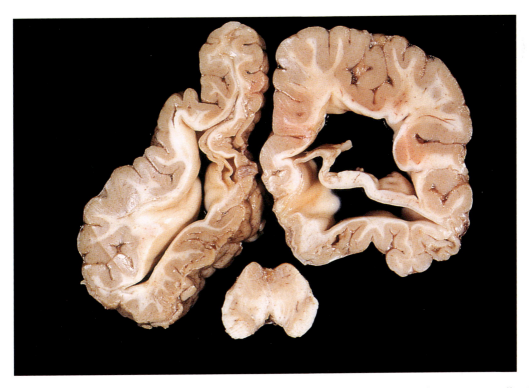

Figure 4.8 Periventricular leukomalacia. Gross appearance of the cerebrum shows that the damage principally affects the white matter adjacent to the ventricles, resulting in periventricular loss and cavity formation

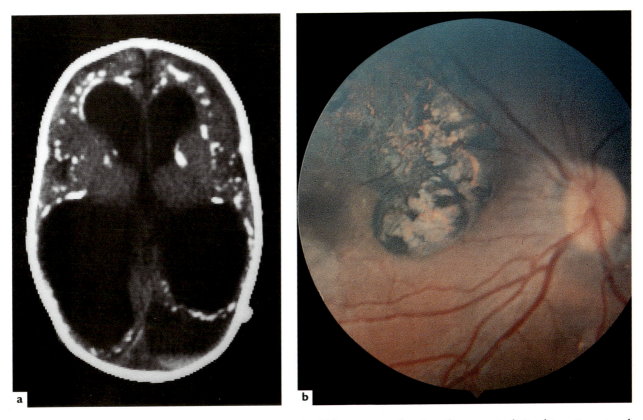

Figure 4.9 Congenital *Toxoplasma* infection. A 10-month-old boy presented with epilepsy, cortical visual impairment and developmental delay due to congenital *Toxoplasma* infection. Axial CT (a) shows ventriculomegaly (hydrocephalus) and diffuse periventricular calcification; funduscopy (b) reveals gross pigmented chorioretinitis

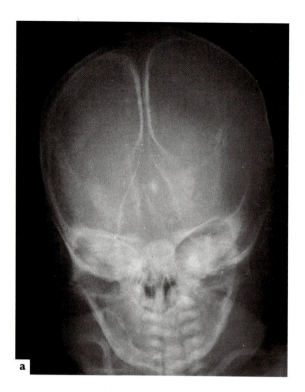
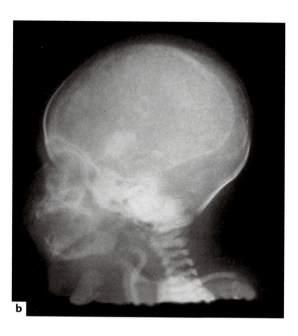

Figure 4.10 Congenital cytomegalovirus (CMV) infection. A 4-day-old girl presented with microcephaly, retinal scarring (see Figure 4.11), and frequent tonic and myoclonic seizures due to congenital CMV infection. Anteroposterior (a) and lateral (b) X-rays of the skull show ventriculomegaly and marked, almost continuous, periventricular calcification

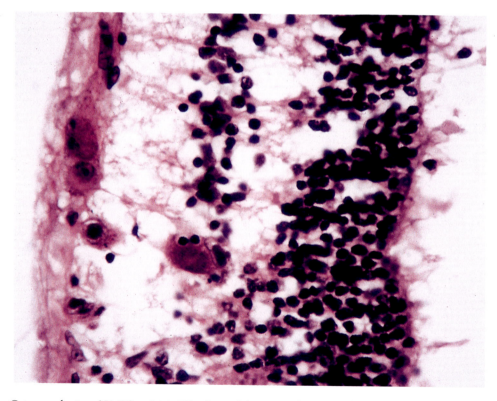

Figure 4.11 Cytomegalovirus (CMV) retinitis. Histology of the retina shows ganglion cells to contain large intranuclear and smaller granular intracytoplasmic CMV inclusion bodies. (H & E)

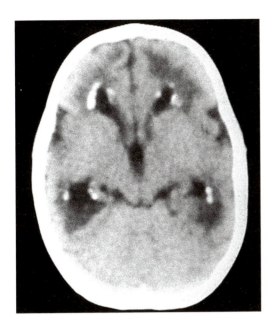

Figure 4.12 Congenital cytomegalovirus (CMV) infection. A 3-month-old infant presented with microcephaly, and myoclonic and tonic seizures due to congenital CMV infection. Axial non-contrast CT shows periventricular calcification and probable major neuronal migration abnormalities (pachygyria)

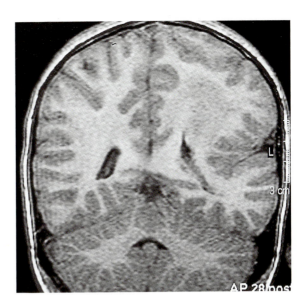

Figure 4.14 Hemimegalencephaly. A 9-year-old child with a mild right hemiparesis diagnosed at 13 months of age who then developed partial and rare secondarily generalized tonic-clonic seizures from 20 months of age. Coronal, T1-weighted MRI shows left hemimegalencephaly with an extensive neuronal migration defect (pachygyria and abnormal configuration of the left perisylvian region)

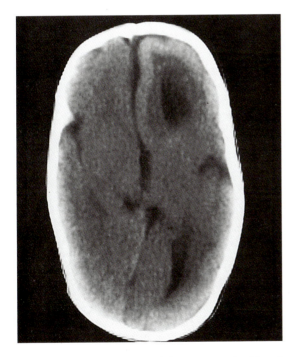

Figure 4.13 Hemimegalencephaly. A 3-week-old infant boy, who presented with drug-resistant intractable seizures, was 'cured' by a left hemispherectomy. Axial CT shows left hemimegalencephaly, and left frontal cortical thickening with pachygyria, prominence of the cortical sulci and dilatation of the left lateral ventricle

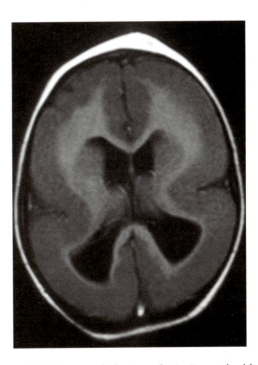

Figure 4.15 Lissencephaly type 1. A 3-month-old girl with lissencephaly due to Miller-Dieker syndrome. The diagnosis of lissencephaly ('smooth brain') was identified on fetal ultrasonography at 30 weeks' gestation and subsequently confirmed on MRI and chromosomal analysis at 3 months of age. Myoclonic and subtle tonic seizures had developed at 2 months of age

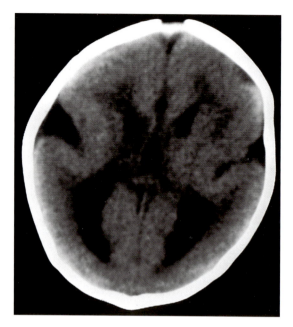

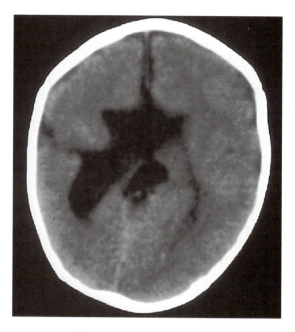

Figure 4.16 Type I lissencephaly. A 6-week-old boy presented with microcephaly and frequent seizures from birth. Axial CT shows a smooth cortex with an interface between gray and white matter, a thick cortical mantle and a lack of an operculum with open sylvian fissures

Figure 4.18 Schizencephaly. A 6-month-old boy presented with developmental delay, cortical visual impairment and infantile spasms. Axial CT shows a major cerebral malformation with unilateral schizencephaly, agenesis of the corpus callosum and an abnormal white–gray matter differentiation, particularly within the left frontal lobe

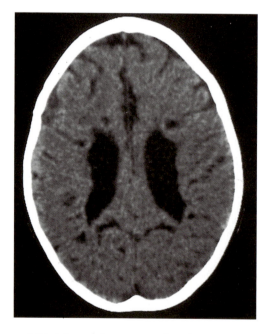

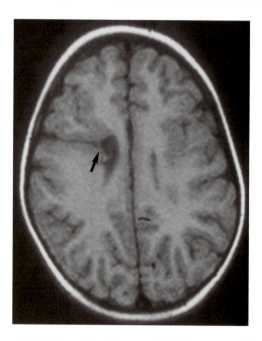

Figure 4.17 Neuronal migration disorder. A 3½-year-old girl presented with persistent seizures, and repeated episodes of convulsive and non-convulsive status epilepticus from age 1 week. Axial CT shows irregular dysmorphic lateral ventricles (probably due to heterotopic gray matter), deep sulci and no discernible white–gray matter differentiation

Figure 4.19 Open-lip schizencephaly. A 22-year-old man with infrequent but drug-resistant partial seizures and a subtle left hemiparesis. Axial, T1-weighted MRI shows a right open-lip schizencephaly with heterotopic gray matter lining the cleft. The cleft opens directly into the enlarged and dysmorphic lateral ventricle; (at this level there is a thin ribbon of gray matter between the cleft and lateral ventricle (arrow) that was absent on contiguous (more caudal) slices)

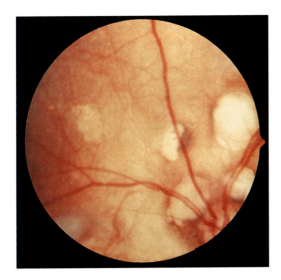

Figure 4.20 Aicardi syndrome. A 2-year-old girl presented with infantile spasms, frequent partial seizures, profound learning difficulties, cerebral dysgenesis, vertebral abnormalities and chorioretinopathy. Fundoscopy shows numerous 'punched-out', hypopigmented retinal lacunae, characteristic of Aicardi syndrome chorioretinopathy. Both lobar and alobar (see Figure 4.26) holoprosencephaly may occur. However, the most commonly found malformation in Aicardi syndrome is agenesis of the corpus callosum (see Figures 4.21–4.23)

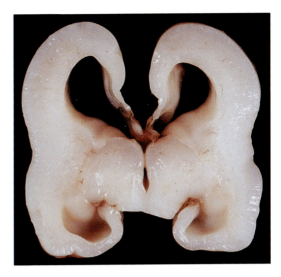

Figure 4.22 Agenesis of the corpus callosum in a fetus (at approximately week 16 of gestation). The corpus callosum is completely absent. The ventricles are dilated and the hippocampi are poorly formed

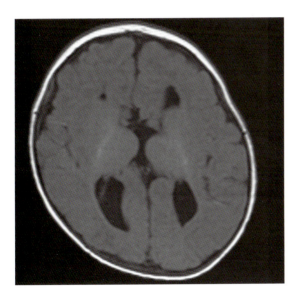

Figure 4.21 Agenesis of the corpus callosum. A 5-month-old girl with global developmental delay apparent from 6–8 weeks of age; infantile spasms developed from 5 months of age and were resistant to medication. Fundoscopy revealed unilateral hypopigmented retinal lacunae. Axial T1-weighted MRI shows agenesis of the corpus callosum, as shown by free communication between the interhemispheric fissure and third ventricle. There is moderate dilatation of the occipital horns of the lateral ventricles

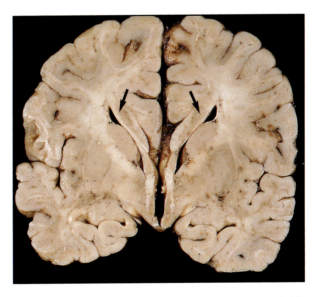

Figure 4.23 Agenesis of the corpus callosum in a child. The agenesis is complete, and Probst bundles are conspicuous (arrowed)

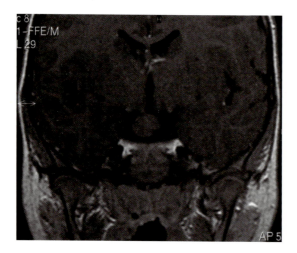

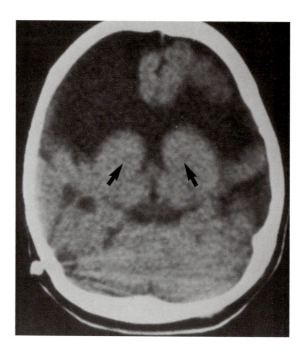

Figure 4.24 Hypothalamic hamartoma. A 17-year-old woman presented with recurrent episodes that had been occurring all of her life. These had previously been diagnosed as being 'behavioral'. She would have a stereotyped warning that she found difficult to describe, and then laugh uncontrollably for about 15 s. These episodes would occur on a daily basis. She had never had a tonic-clonic seizure. She was diagnosed as having gelastic seizures, and subsequent MRI scan showed evidence of a hypothalamic hamartoma

Figure 4.25 Semilobar/alobar holoprosencephaly. A 6-month-old infant with microcephaly, mid-face hypoplasia and myoclonic seizures. Axial CT showing an 'island' of cortex in the frontal lobes (left > right), a holoventricle and partially separated thalami (arrows)

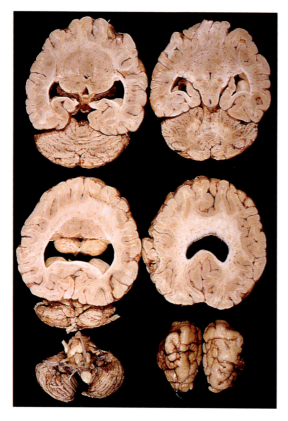

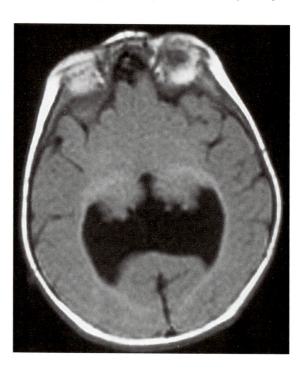

Figure 4.26 Holoprosencephaly (alobar). Multiple coronal sections of the brain reveal only a rudimentary interhemispheric fissure, a large single ventricle and fusion of the deep gray nuclei

Figure 4.27 Semilobar holoprosencephaly. A 4-month-old infant with microcephaly, hypotonia, feeding problems and frequent 'subtle' seizures ('cycling' and 'boxing' movements). Axial T1-weighted MRI shows a single, large telencephalic ventricle which is in continuity with a small third ventricle. The posterior part of the interhemispheric fissure is present and the gyral pattern suggests pachygyria

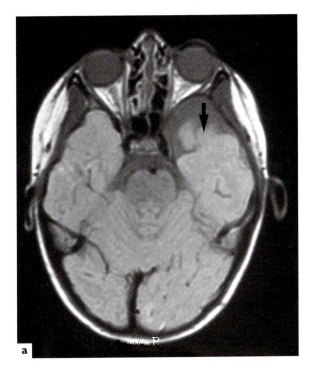
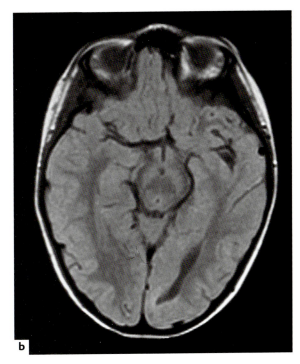

Figure 4.28 Temporal lobe agenesis. A 6-year-old girl had frequent, brief, simple and complex partial seizures that were controlled by antiepileptic drugs. MRI scans show partial agenesis of the left temporal lobe (a; arrow), and dysgenesis of the left temporal and occipital lobes (b)

NEURODEGENERATIVE AND METABOLIC ENCEPHALOPATHIES

A number of rare age-related neurodegenerative conditions (Figure 4.29), including some inherited metabolic disorders, cause seizures and epilepsy. The clinical picture is usually progressive myoclonic epilepsy with or without dementia (Table 4.1).

Mitochondrial cytopathies

These form a heterogeneous group of multisystem diseases with diverse clinical presentations; the only common factor is a non-specific morphological finding on muscle biopsy – the 'ragged red' fiber (Figure 4.30). Myoclonic epilepsy with ragged red fibers (MERRF) usually presents in adolescence/early adulthood, but may occur at any age (Figure 4.31). Myoclonus, tonic-clonic seizures, muscle weakness and ataxia are prominent features. This phenotype is most frequently associated with maternal inheritance and has been linked to a point mutation of the transfer RNA lysine gene. Neonatal seizures may also be caused by a mitochondrial cytopathy. Mitochondrial encephalopathy with lactic acidosis and stroke-

like episodes (MELAS) is a mitochondrial cytopathy that typically presents with stroke-like episodes before the age of 40 and an encephalopathy which is characterized by seizures (often myoclonic) or dementia (or both) (Figure 4.32).

Lipidoses

These are a heterogeneous group of conditions characterized by accumulation of lipid-containing materials in neurons and other cells due to inherited lysosomal enzyme defects. A juvenile-onset form is characterized by extreme stimulus-sensitive myoclonus, generalized tonic-clonic seizures, dementia, rigidity, pseudobulbar palsy and, ultimately, quadriplegia. Rectal (Figure 4.33) and skin biopsies are useful methods of diagnosing lysosomal deficiency affecting the central nervous system.

Baltic myoclonus

This autosomal recessive condition has a peak age of onset at 10 years. The epilepsy is characterized by stimulus-sensitive myoclonus and generalized tonic-clonic seizures, both of which are usually well

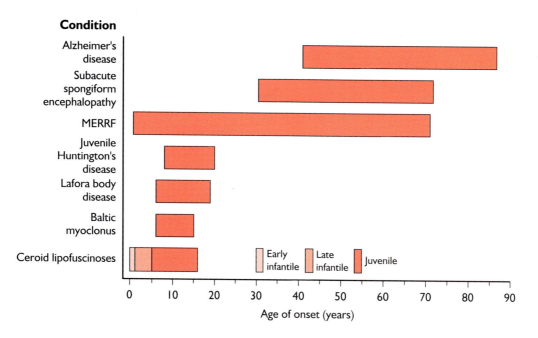

Figure 4.29 Age of onset of some of the rare neurodegenerative conditions causing seizures and epilepsy

Table 4.1 Disorders in which clinical presentation is either typically or occasionally progressive myoclonic epilepsy

---

Typically progressive myoclonic epilepsy

Lafora's body disease

Ramsay Hunt syndrome (dyssynergia cerebellaris myoclonica)

Sialidosis type 1 (cherry-red spot myoclonus syndrome)

Sialidosis type 2

Mucolipidosis type 1

Juvenile neuropathic Gaucher's disease (type 3)

Juvenile neuroaxonal dystrophy

Occasionally progressive myoclonic epilepsy

Ceroid lipofuscinoses

    early and late infantile forms

    early and late juvenile forms

Myoclonic epilepsy with ragged red fibers (MERRF)

Huntington's disease

Wilson's disease

Hallervorden–Spatz disease

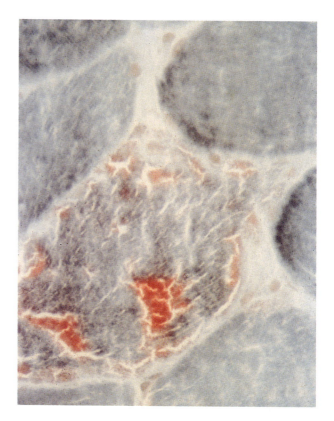

Figure 4.30 'Ragged red' fibers. A 27-year-old man developed a progressive illness comprising ataxia, myoclonic epilepsy and dementia, which culminated in death after 5 years. Histology of the central fiber in a frozen muscle section shows coarse red staining, indicative of abnormalities of mitochondrial distribution, structure and function. (Gomori trichrome)

controlled with sodium valproate. Survival into adult life is common and the prognosis is much more favorable than previously recognized. Dementia does not occur, although the use of phenytoin may be associated with a significant decline in cognitive function.

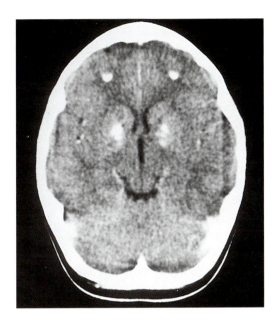

Figure 4.31 Myoclonic epilepsy with ragged red fibers (MERRF). A 14-year-old boy presented with short stature, learning difficulties and epilepsy (myoclonic and generalized tonic-clonic seizures). Non-contrast axial CT shows symmetrical areas of calcification within the basal ganglia and frontal lobes. (Serum and cerebrospinal fluid showed high levels of lactate, and muscle biopsy revealed ragged red fibers)

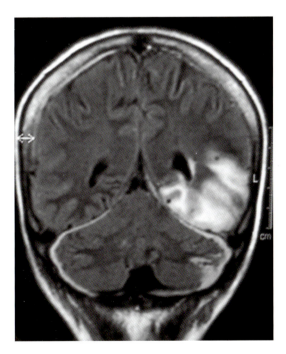

Figure 4.32 Mitochondrial encephalopathy with lactic acidosis and stroke-like episodes (MELAS). Post-contrast T1-weighted MRI showing cortical enhancement in a recent posterior circulation infarct in a patient with proven MELAS. Note also the leptomeningeal enhancement which can be seen post-lumbar puncture as in this patient

Lafora body disease

This autosomal recessive condition is manifested by stimulus-sensitive myoclonus, generalized tonic-clonic seizures and partial seizures with visual auras. Onset is during late childhood/adolescence. The clinical course involves progressive dementia, dysarthria and ataxia until death in the teens or early twenties. Pathologically, the condition is characterized by neuronal inclusions (Lafora bodies; Figure 4.34) in the cerebellar cortex, brain stem nucleus and spinal cord.

Huntington's disease

This is characterized by the triad of dominant inheritance, choreoathetosis and progressive dementia. The responsible genetic defect is a trinucleotide expansion on the short arm of the fourth chromosome. The juvenile-onset form (Westphal variant) frequently presents with bradykinesia, rigidity and ataxia, and is associated with seizures in 50% of cases. The adult-onset form is occasionally complicated by a seizure disorder. The CT (Figure 4.35) and postmortem findings (Figures 4.36 and 4.37) are striking.

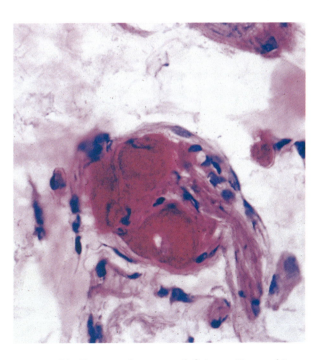

Figure 4.33 Lysosomal enzyme deficiency. Frozen histological section of rectal biopsy shows the cytoplasm of ganglion cells in the myenteric plexus to be distended by strongly PAS-positive glycolipid. (Periodic Acid–Schiff)

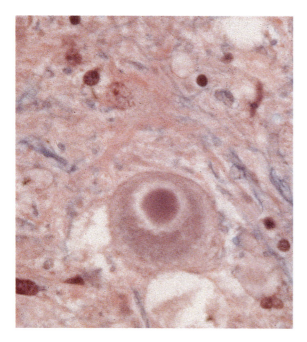

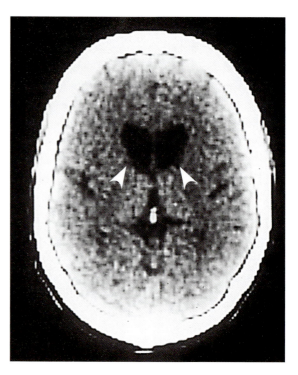

Figure 4.34 Lafora body disease. A postmortem was carried out on a teenage gypsy girl with an undiagnosed progressive neurological disorder. She had never been investigated by a neurologist and was found dead in her caravan. This neuron, from the dorsal horn of the spinal cord, contains a large Lafora body in the perikaryon showing the typical central dense zone and lucent halo. The bodies consist of polyglucosan material. (H & E–luxol-fast blue)

Figure 4.35 Huntington's disease. A 51-year-old woman presented with dementia, myoclonus and 'restlessness'. Non-contrast axial CT shows the loss of the normal bulge in the inferolateral border of the frontal horn of the lateral ventricle (arrowed). There is also diffuse enlargement of the lateral ventricles

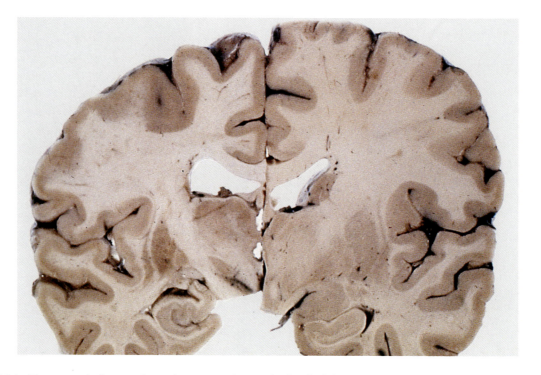

Figure 4.36 Huntington's disease. Coronal sections taken at the level of the pes hippocampi of a normal cerebrum (right side) and a cerebrum showing the pathological changes of Huntington's disease (left side), namely, near-complete atrophy of the caudate nucleus and, to a lesser extent, of the lentiform nucleus, particularly the putamen

Subacute spongiform encephalopathy (Creutzfeldt–Jakob disease)

The sporadic form of this disease typically presents in middle age, but it may occur in young adults. In humans, transmission has been through corneal transplants, depth electrodes and human growth hormone injections. It is transmitted by a prion protein. After a latency period of 20–30 years (sometimes less), a rapidly progressive dementia ensues, culminating in death in less than a year. The EEG evolves into a characteristic pattern (Figure 4.38) and MRI may show abnormal high signal in the basal ganglia on T2-weighted images (Figure 4.39). CSF may be positive for the 14-3-3 brain protein but false positive and negative results may occur. The histopathological features are unique (Figure 4.40).

Variant CJD has been recognized since the mid-1990s, mainly in the UK, and is now known to result from ingestion of food products infected with bovine spongiform encephalopathy (BSE). Most commonly variant CJD presents in younger patients than in the sporadic form of the disease and frequently has a neuropsychiatric presentation, with anxiety, depression and widespread sensory symptoms being com-mon early features. Seizures may occur, and can mimic myoclonic epilepsy. There is an inevitable progressive ataxia and dementia with death usually within 2 years of onset. EEG changes are not charac-teristic, but magnetic resonance imaging (MRI) may reveal the typical 'pulvinar sign' of high signal in the pulvinar nucleus of the thalamus (Figure 4.41).

Alzheimer's disease

This is the most common of the neurodegenerative conditions. It usually commences in the seventh decade, although a familial, dominantly inherited, form occurs in mid-life. The onset is insidious and the course slowly progressive, with deterioration of memory, personality, language and, ultimately, motor function leading to death within 5–15 years. Alzheimer's disease is associated with a 10-fold increased risk of epilepsy compared with an age-matched population, and 15% experience seizures 10 years after diagnosis. Diffuse cerebral atrophy is visible on cerebral imaging (Figure 4.42) and the his-tological appearances are classical (Figures 4.43 and 4.44).

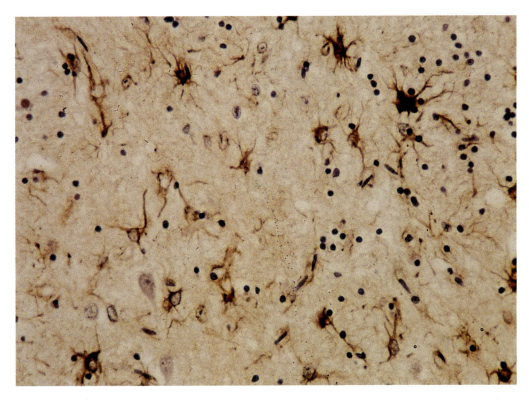

Figure 4.37 Huntington's disease. Histology of the caudate nucleus shows marked loss of small- and medium-sized neurons, and proliferation of large reactive GFAP-positive astrocytes. (Immunoperoxidase method for glial fibrillary acidic protein (GFAP))

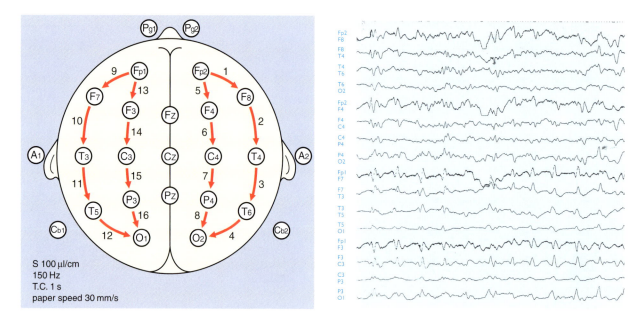

Figure 4.38 Sporadic Creutzfeldt–Jakob disease. A 62-year-old woman, first seen by a neurologist in a psychiatric unit, initially presented with paranoid ideation, followed by a rapid progressive decline in cognitive function. Examination revealed ataxia, quadriparesis, cortical blindness and multifocal myoclonus. Her EEGs show a diffuse background slow-wave abnormality with relative impoverishment over the left hemisphere and frequent generalized periodic complexes

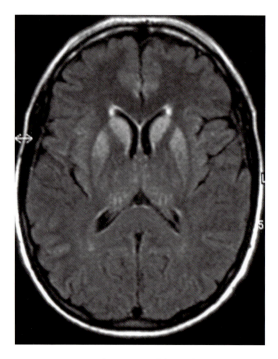

Figure 4.39 Sporadic Creutzfeldt–Jakob disease. MRI FLAIR sequence shows high signal in the caudate nuclei and putamen bilaterally

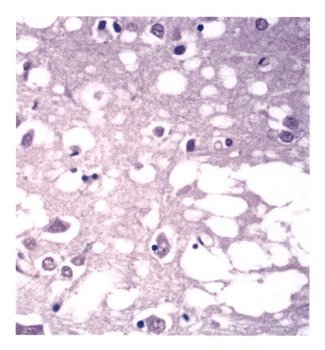

Figure 4.40 Sporadic Creutzfeldt–Jakob disease (subacute spongiform encephalopathy). Histology of the cerebral cortex shows the characteristic spongiform change affecting the neuropil between and adjacent to neurons. Two areas of confluent spongy change are particularly conspicuous in this section. In the later stages of the disease, neuronal loss and gliosis can readily be appreciated (not seen here; H & E)

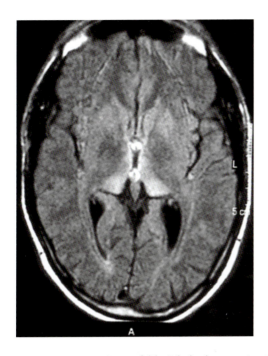

Figure 4.41 Variant Creutzfeldt–Jakob disease. An 18-year-old man initially presented to a psychiatrist with depression and anxiety, but within 4 months he had developed significant ataxia and cognitive slowing. MRI FLAIR sequence shows the 'pulvinar sign' – high signal in the pulvinar nucleus of the posterior thalamus bilaterally

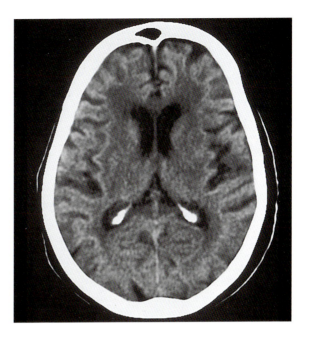

Figure 4.42 Alzheimer's disease. A 65-year-old woman was brought to a neurology outpatients department by her family, who reported a gradual deterioration of memory over the previous 2 years. Examination revealed disorientation in time and place, and a marked expressive dysphasia. Her CT reveals generalized cerebral atrophy with marked widening of the cortical sulci

Reye's syndrome

This syndrome is a rare metabolic encephalopathy associated with the use of salicylic acid (aspirin), although a number of inborn errors of metabolism may also present with a picture resembling Reye's syndrome. Infants and young children present with repeated vomiting, fever, a disturbed conscious level and generalized convulsions. Most children have hypoglycemia and elevated concentrations of serum transaminases. There may be a prodromal viral illness, and different stages (or levels) of coma have been recognized. The mortality rate is high with death due (usually) to severe cerebral edema. The liver shows fatty infiltration, which resolves in survivors (Figure 4.45). Survivors also show varying degrees of neurological impairment and epilepsy.

Neurocutaneous syndromes

These constitute a collection of hereditary diseases caused by an unknown defect that affects structures of ectodermal origin. The syndromes are characterized by malformations and tumors in numerous organs, but notably in the skin, eye and nervous system. Three of the more common syndromes associated with epilepsy are described below.

Tuberous sclerosis

This is transmitted as an autosomal dominant trait with incomplete penetrance which is strongly associated with male gender. The principal manifestations are mental retardation, seizures, skin lesions and tumors.

The classical cutaneous malformation is adenoma sebaceum (Figure 4.46). Additional cutaneous features include shagreen patches (Figure 4.47), periungual fibromata (Figure 4.48) and depigmented ash-leaf patches. The earliest sign may be a fibrous plaque on the forehead (Figure 4.49). Epilepsy is invariable in learning-impaired individuals and usual in the remainder. Tuberous sclerosis is a relatively common cause of infantile spasms; later presentation is in the form of partial or generalized seizures. Tuberous sclerosis must be excluded in any child under 18 months of age who presents with both infantile spasms and partial seizures.

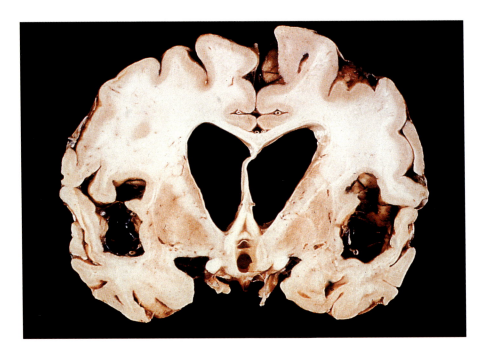

Figure 4.43 Alzheimer's disease. Coronal section of the cerebrum at the level of the mammillary bodies shows severe cerebral atrophy, most noticeably in the superior temporal gyri, with widening of the fissures, particularly the sylvian fissures, and marked dilatation of the lateral and third ventricles. In patients with Alzheimer's disease, the brain rarely manifests such a severe degree of atrophy at the time of death

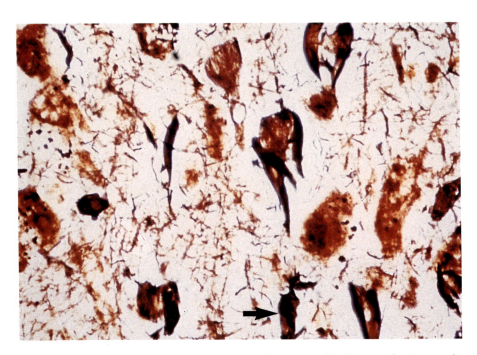

Figure 4.44 Alzheimer's disease. Histology of the hippocampus shows neurofibrillary tangles (arrowed) in virtually every large neuron. (von Braunmuhl's silver-impregnation technique)

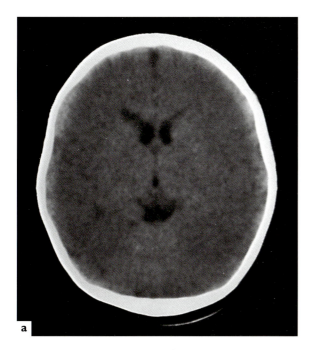
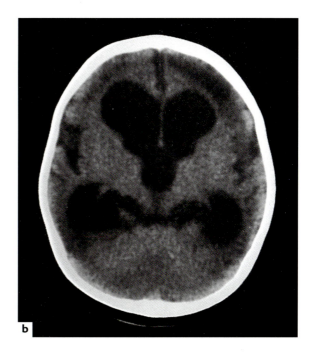

Figure 4.45 Reye's syndrome. A 7-month-old girl developed severe neurological impairment and intractable epilepsy following Reye's syndrome. Axial CTs show obliteration of normal white–gray matter differentiation (diffuse low-density pattern) at presentation (a), and 2 months later, obstructive hydrocephalus (b)

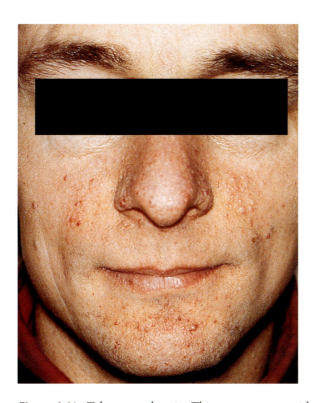

Figure 4.46 Tuberous sclerosis. This young man with tuberous sclerosis had well-controlled complex partial seizures. Multiple angiofibromas (adenoma sebaceum) are especially prominent in the nasolabial folds

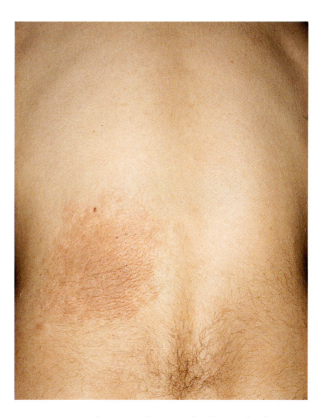

Figure 4.47 Tuberous sclerosis. The lower back (same patient as in Figure 4.46) reveals a large shagreen patch

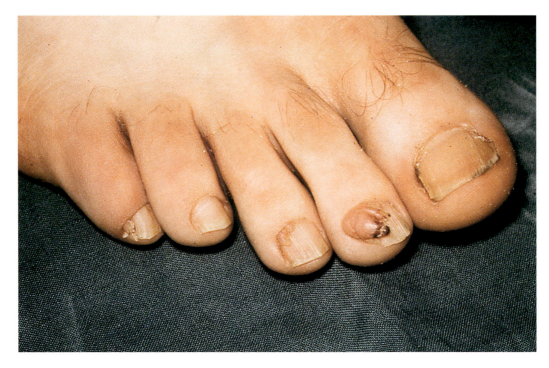

Figure 4.48 Tuberous sclerosis. Periungual fibromas, shown here on the foot (same patient as in Figures 4.46 and 4.47) may be the only cutaneous manifestation of tuberous sclerosis. Thus, the feet should always be examined if this diagnosis is suspected – including in the parents of children whose epilepsy is caused by tuberous sclerosis

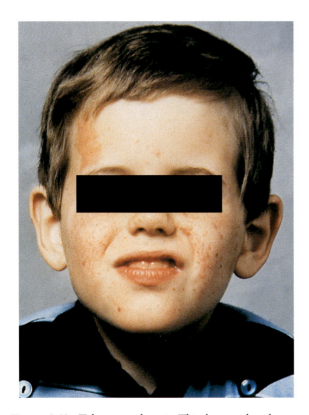

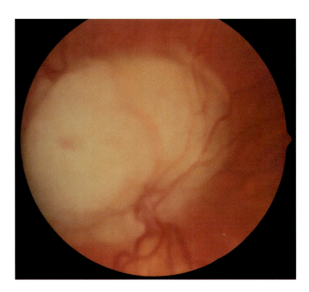

Figure 4.50 Tuberous sclerosis. Funduscopy shows a large pale retinal tumor

Figure 4.49 Tuberous sclerosis. This boy with tuberous sclerosis has myoclonic and partial seizures. Angiofibromas (adenoma sebaceum) and a fibrous plaque are seen on the right forehead

Benign cerebral, retinal (Figure 4.50) and renal tumors are found in 15%, 50% and 80% of cases, respectively. Malignant cerebral tumors can also develop, typically a subependymal giant cell astrocytoma (SEGA) (Figure 4.51). Cardiac involvement with rhabdomyomata may be demonstrated on

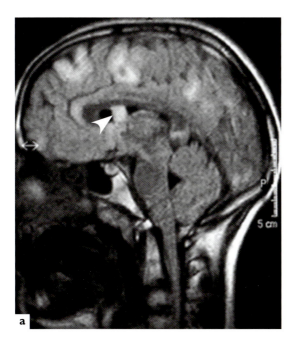

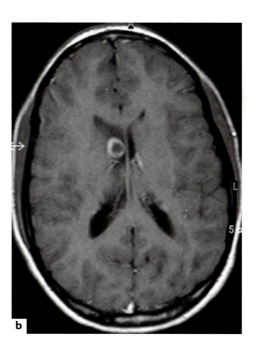

Figure 4.51 Tuberous sclerosis. A 22-year-old man with tuberous sclerosis and a 5-year history of partial and secondarily generalized tonic-clonic seizures and learning difficulties. Parasagittal (a) and axial (b) MRI show a subependymal giant cell astrocytoma (SEGA) (arrow on left parasagittal image); multiple hyperintense cortical lesions also seen on the left parasagittal image)

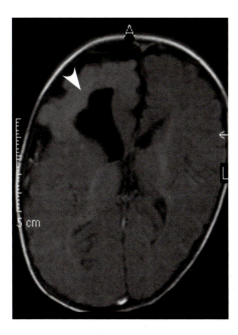

Figure 4.52 Tuberous sclerosis. Axial T1-weighted MRI in a 9-month-old infant with global developmental delay and intractable focal seizures and infantile spasms shows a grossly dysplastic and thickened right frontal lobe (arrow) with less obvious dysplastic changes affecting the rest of the right cerebral hemisphere. The child demonstrated an over 90% reduction in seizures after a right frontal and anterior parietal lobectomy undertaken at 17 months of age

routine antenatal (fetal) ultrasonography and typically provides the first clue that the child has tuberous sclerosis. The tubers are areas of gliosis within the cerebral hemispheres in which extensive calcification results in a classical appearance on CT scanning. Additional cerebral dysgenesis (cortical dysplasia) (Figure 4.52) is frequently seen in tuberous sclerosis particularly with MRI.

Sturge–Weber syndrome (encephalotrigeminal angiomatosis)

The full syndrome comprises a port-wine vascular nevus on the face, generalized or focal contralateral hemiparesis or homonymous hemianopia, ipsilateral intracranial calcification and mental retardation. The cutaneous angioma (Figure 4.53) is evident at birth and may extend to the pharynx or other viscera. Ninety per cent of cases develop seizures in the first year of life; hemiparesis occurs in 30–40% and mental retardation in 80%.

The leptomeningeal angiomatosis has a propensity for the occipital or occipitoparietal regions. Cortical calcification underlying the vascular malformation is evident on skull X-ray (Figure 4.54) and CT scanning (Figures 4.55 and 4.56). Both the leptomeningeal angiomatosis and the hemiparesis

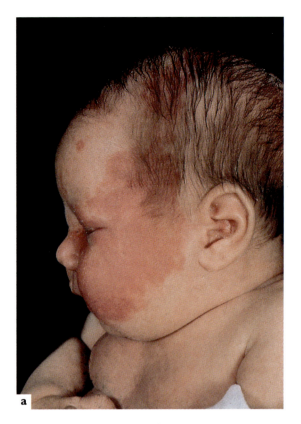

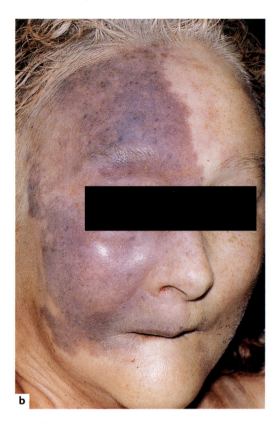

Figure 4.53 Sturge–Weber syndrome. Cutaneous angiomata seen in an infant (a) and in an adult (b)

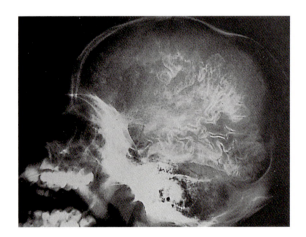

Figure 4.54 Sturge–Weber syndrome. In an 8-year-old girl with persistent partial seizures due to this neurocutaneous syndrome, a plain lateral skull X-ray shows diffuse, mainly parieto-occipital 'railroad track' or 'tramline' calcification, characteristic of the venous malformation in this syndrome

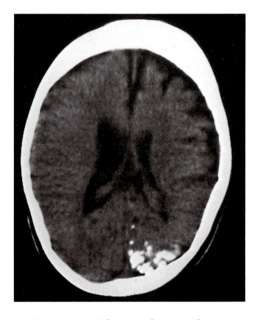

Figure 4.55 Sturge–Weber syndrome. This 15-year-old girl has an extensive facial nevus with intra-esophageal extension, left hemiparesis, intractable epilepsy and moderate mental handicap. CT shows right hemisphere atrophy with occipital calcification. A year after right hemispherectomy, the patient was seizure-free with significant improvements in both behavior and cognition

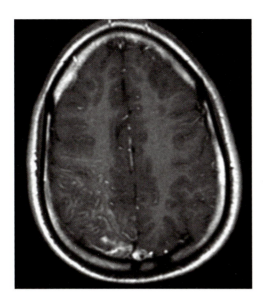

Figure 4.56 Sturge–Weber syndrome. An 18-year-old woman with Sturge–Weber syndrome and infrequent partial seizures affecting only the left side of her body with rare secondarily generalized tonic-clonic seizures. Axial, post-contrast MRI shows thickening of the diploic space bilaterally, abnormal enhancement in the right occipital cortex suggesting calcification in superficial cortical veins and subtle atrophy of the right occipital lobe

progress over time and in view of this 'early' hemispherectomy or hemispherotomy is generally considered as the treatment of choice.

Neurofibromatosis (NF)

This dominantly inherited condition takes two forms: NF I (central) and NF II (peripheral). It is the most common single-gene defect affecting the central nervous system, with an incidence of 1 in 2000 population. Cutaneous lesions include café-au-lait spots (Figure 4.57), plexiform neurofibromata, axillary freckling and subcutaneous fibromata. Individuals usually have relative or absolute megalencephaly and some degree of learning difficulty. Seizures occur in 10–15% of patients with NF I and are often associated with intracranial tumors (Figure 4.58), or other lesions that may be seen in both the cortex and thalami and which may be either symmetric or asymmetric.

INFECTIONS

Infections of the central nervous system account for 2–3% of all cases of epilepsy, but are among the most

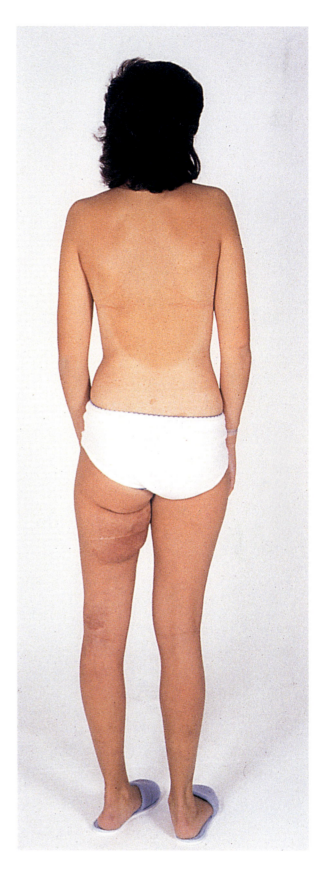

Figure 4.57 Neurofibromatosis. Café-au-lait spots are present on the trunk and neurofibromata can be seen on the posterior aspect of the left leg

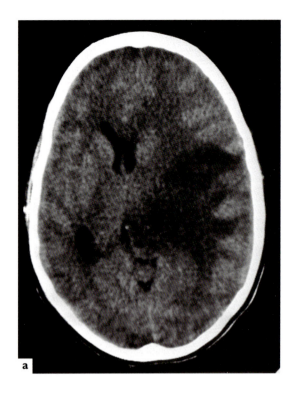

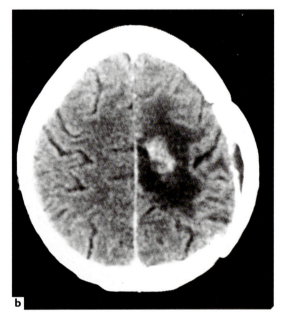

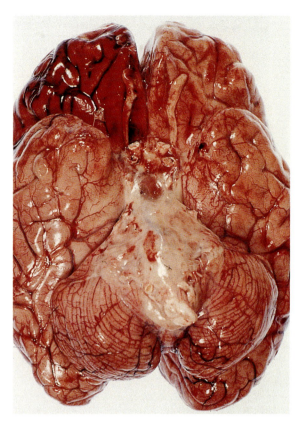

Figure 4.59 Bacterial meningitis. A 65-year-old male alcoholic was found unconscious in a park. Cerebrospinal fluid examination was consistent with pneumococcal meningitis. Despite appropriate therapy, he died within 48 h. The postmortem examination confirmed acute bacterial leptomeningitis. The base of the brain shows copious amounts of pus in the subarachnoid space over the brain stem and cerebellum, and in the interpeduncular fossa. The right frontal lobe shows early hemorrhagic infarction

Figure 4.58 Neurofibromatosis. A 12-year-old girl with type I neurofibromatosis presented with a progressive mild right hemiparesis and two right-sided focal motor-onset, secondarily generalized, seizures. Non-contrast axial CT (a) shows marked edema of the left hemisphere with mid-line shift, and compression of the frontal and occipital horns of the left lateral ventricle. CT at a higher level, with contrast (b), reveals an irregular but well-defined mass within the area of edema. An astrocytoma (grade 1) was completely removed at operation. The patient experienced no further seizures at follow-up 2 years later

common causes in infants and preschool children. The risk of developing epilepsy and its subsequent prognosis depend on the severity of the illness and the age at which infection occurs.

Bacterial meningitis

The 20-year risk of later epilepsy is 13.4% if the acute illness is complicated by seizures and 2.4% if it is not. The apparently higher risk associated with certain organisms is probably due to their occurrence in younger children. Poor prognostic factors include extremes of age, bacteremia, seizures, coma, concomitant systemic illness and delayed treatment (Figures 4.59 and 4.60).

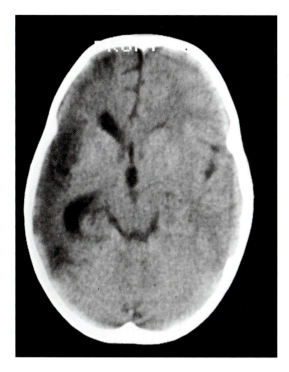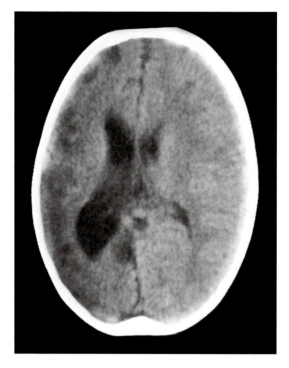

Figure 4.60 Bacterial meningitis. In a 4½-year-old girl with right hemiparesis, and partial and secondarily generalized seizures following meningococcal meningitis, axial CTs show infarction of the left hemisphere with consequent 'atrophy' and ventricular enlargement; she developed partial and secondarily generalized seizures that responded to a single antiepileptic drug

Cerebral abscess

Cerebral abscess is virtually always secondary to a suppurative process elsewhere in the body. The source may be within the skull (40%), metastatic (33%), or unidentified (20%). Effective antibiotic therapy and improvements in ear, nose and throat surgery have reduced the incidence of abscesses secondary to sinus or middle ear disease. The main sources of metastatic abscesses are from the heart (Figure 4.61), lungs and teeth. Clinical presentation is variable with focal and generalized seizures being common. The diagnosis should be considered sooner rather than later, as the earlier the diagnosis and medical treatment, the better the outcome. CT scanning is able to detect abscesses greater than 1 cm in diameter (Figure 4.62).

Initial treatment should be medical, with the choice of antibiotics guided by knowledge of the source of sepsis. Surgical intervention may be necessary if deterioration occurs. The advances in imaging have improved the prognosis, but the clinical course remains unpredictable and the mortality rate is still approximately 20% (Figure 4.63). Focal epilepsy is the most common sequela and the risk rises over

time. On 10-year follow-up, 90% of the patients requiring surgical intervention will have developed this complication.

Subdural empyema

This usually occurs as a consequence of frontal or ethmoidal sinusitis (Figure 4.64) due to direct extension or venous spread of infection. The most common offending pathogens are streptococci.

Focal seizures, due to local cerebral ischemic necrosis, are a late feature associated with a rapidly deteriorating conscious level. CT or MR scanning is diagnostic (Figure 4.65). Urgent surgical drainage is usually required, but the mortality rate is high (Figure 4.66).

Viral encephalitis

Herpes simplex virus (HSV) encephalitis is the most common and most severe form of acute encephalitis. Acute symptomatic seizures and symptoms suggesting temporal lobe involvement are common presenting features. Cerebrospinal fluid (CSF) lymphocytosis is usual, but a high red cell count and

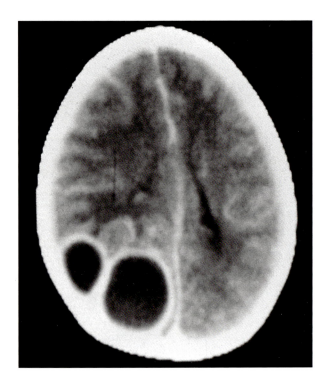

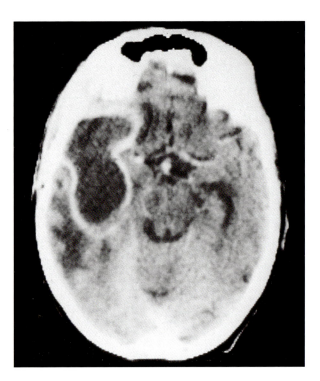

Figure 4.61 Cerebral abscess. A 4-year-old boy with congenital cyanotic heart disease presented with focal seizures and fever. Contrast-enhanced axial CT shows two well-defined ring-enhancing cerebral abscesses within the left occipital lobe, and some mass effect

Figure 4.62 Cerebral abscess. Contrast-enhanced CT shows a large biloculated lesion with an enhancing rim and a lower-density center in the right temporal region with surrounding and more posterior edema

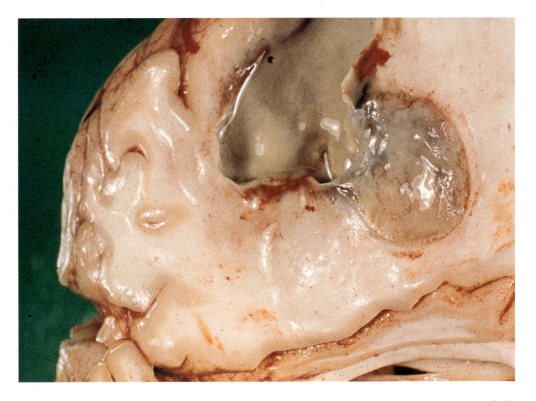

Figure 4.63 Cerebral abscess. Horizontal section through the right frontal lobe shows a large convoluted abscess with a thick fibrous wall containing an abundance of pus

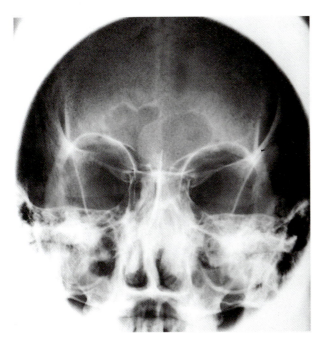

Figure 4.64 Frontal sinusitis with mucocele. Plain skull X-ray shows loss of lucency of the right frontal sinus, the margins of which have lost their normal irregularity and become thinned

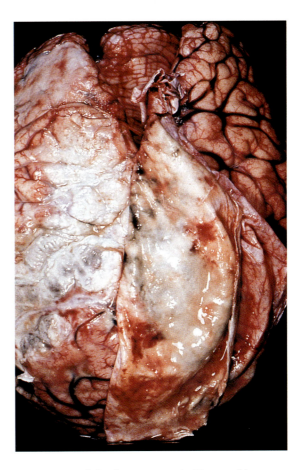

Figure 4.66 Subdural empyema. A 42-year-old man was admitted to hospital with a 5-day history of headache, confusion, left facial twitching and swelling of the right temporoparietal scalp. Examination revealed dysarthria, deviation of eyes and head to the left, and left facial focal motor seizures. There was also spasm of the right temporalis and masseter muscles, and a boggy swelling over the right temporal region. Despite surgical intervention and broad-spectrum antibiotics, death ensued 6 days later. In this view of the brain from above, the dura has been reflected from over the right cerebral hemisphere. There is pus adhering to the inner aspect of the dura as well as covering the right cerebral convexity

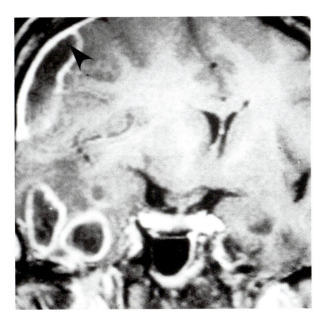

Figure 4.65 Subdural empyema. This enhanced CT shows two ring-enhancing lesions with a lower-density center in the right temporal region. There is a larger extra-axial collection lying superiorly (arrow). The margins are enhanced and the center is of low density. The lower lesions are abscess cavities whereas the uppermost lesion is a subdural empyema

xanthochromia reflect the hemorrhagic nature of the lesions. A polymerase chain reaction (PCR) amplification assay is highly sensitive and specific for the detection of HSV DNA in the CSF of patients with HSV encephalitis. The EEG (Figure 4.67) has a typical appearance, but this is not specific to HSV. In children, the classical EEG appearances may not be seen (Figure 4.68).

CT scanning may show evidence of temporal lobe involvement (Figure 4.69), but this is seen more clearly with MRI (Figure 4.70) and may be useful in

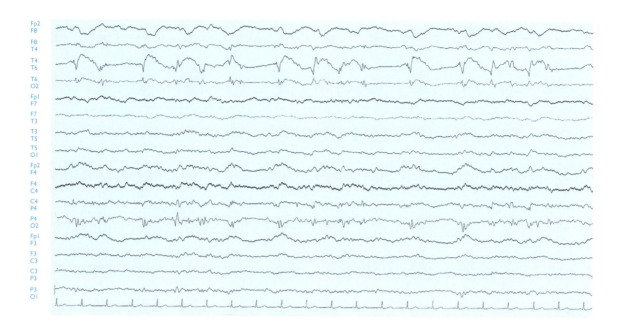

Figure 4.67 Herpes simplex encephalitis. A 62-year-old Cypriot woman had a 4-day history of headache, fever and deterioration of level of consciousness, and two secondarily generalized tonic-clonic seizures. EEG shows 'periodic complexes' – high-voltage sharp waves occurring at 2-s intervals over the right posterior temporal region

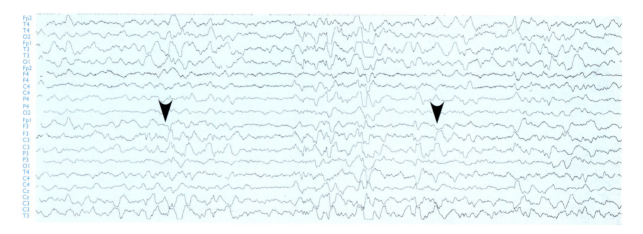

Figure 4.68 Herpes simplex encephalitis. A 7-year-old boy had focal seizures and increasing stupor due to herpes simplex encephalitis. EEG shows bilateral but asymmetrical high-amplitude paroxysmal activity against a slow background. The slow activity predominates over the left hemisphere (arrowed) whereas the right is of relatively low amplitude

differentiating herpes simplex encephalitis from other causes of coma with fever.

As soon as the diagnosis is suspected intravenous acyclovir should be initiated, prior to the investigation with imaging and CSF examination. Cerebral biopsy is rarely indicated (Figure 4.71), particularly since the advent of HSV PCR techniques.

The risk of mortality depends on the age and the level of consciousness at the time of institution of antiviral therapy. Intense hemorrhagic necrosis of the temporal lobe is seen at necropsy (Figure 4.72).

In survivors, neurological sequelae are almost inevitable, the most common of which are amnesic syndromes, dysphasia and temporal lobe epilepsy.

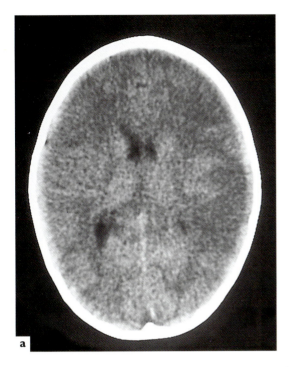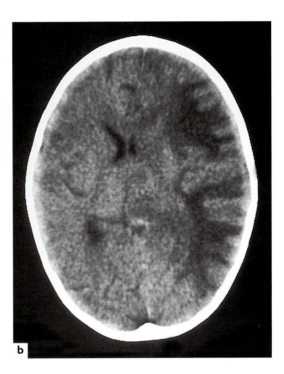

Figure 4.69 Herpes simplex encephalitis. A 2½-year-old boy had a 3-day history of frequent partial and generalized seizures and eventual coma due to herpes simplex encephalitis. Axial CT shows initially a diffuse loss of white–gray matter differentiation and low densities bilaterally, particularly in the right temporoparietal region (a); 10 days later, there was diffuse infarction of the right hemisphere (b)

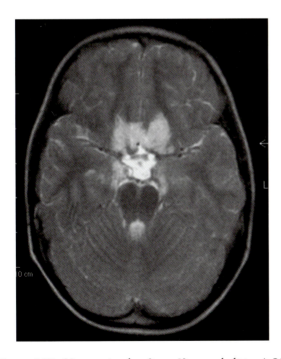

Figure 4.70 Herpes simplex (type 1) encephalitis. A 38-year-old man with a 5-day history of confusion and generalized tonic-clonic seizures. EEG showed bilateral periodic lateralized epileptiform discharges (BiPLEDS). Axial T1-weighted MRI shows bilateral swelling and hyperintensity of both medial temporal lobes with spread into the medial and inferior frontal lobes

The 20-year risk of epilepsy is twice as great if acute symptomatic seizures occur (22% vs. 10%), which is higher than after bacterial meningitis presumably because of direct cerebral parenchymal damage.

Other viral encephalitidies can present similarly, with the specific virus dependent on the geographical location. In Europe, particularly in children, enteroviruses such as echovirus and coxsackie virus are common causes of viral encephalitis. Some of the most common viruses causing encephalitis worldwide are arboviruses, including the flaviviruses Japanese encephalitis (in Asia), West Nile virus (mainly in Africa, Asia and North America) and St Louis encephalitis (North America).

HIV and *Toxoplasma* infection

Human immunodeficiency virus (HIV) infection and the acquired immune deficiency syndrome (AIDS) have reached pandemic proportions. Neurological manifestations are commonly seen and may be due to direct viral invasion or be secondary to immunosuppression. Seizures occur in 10–20% of unselected populations of patients with HIV infection. These are generalized in 75% of cases, but partial-onset seizures may occur in the absence of

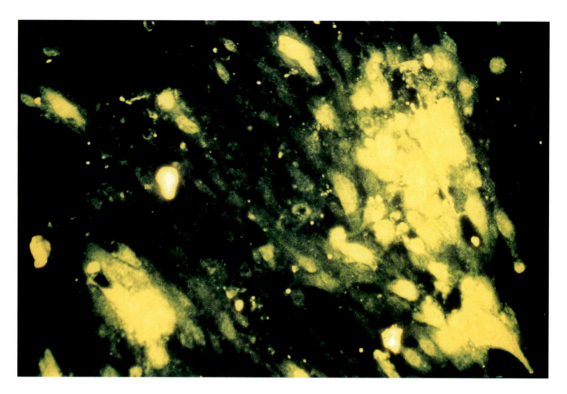

Figure 4.71 Herpes simplex encephalitis. Immunofluorescence of the temporal lobe reveals the presence of fluorescent-labelled antibody and, therefore, abundant herpes simplex antigen. This is one of many reliable methods for diagnosing herpes simplex infection of brain tissue

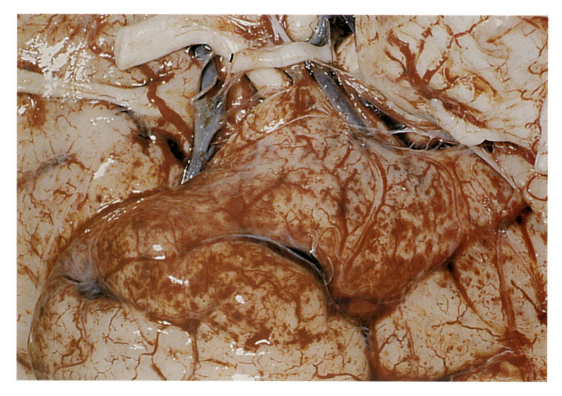

Figure 4.72 Herpes simplex encephalitis. The base of the right brain shows an area of hemorrhagic necrosis affecting the right uncus and adjacent parts of the temporal lobe. This location and appearance are typical of acute herpes simplex encephalitis

focal structural pathology. Both convulsive and non-convulsive status have been reported. Of those with seizures, 15% are seropositive only, 15% have AIDS-related complex and 70% have full-blown AIDS.

Generalized seizures are a common late feature of the AIDS–dementia complex, probably due to progressive cortical damage. Convulsive status, which is associated with a poor prognosis, may simply reflect late severe AIDS. The EEG is usually abnormal, but specific epileptiform features are unusual and, with the exception of non-convulsive status, the EEG rarely yields additional useful clinical information.

Cerebral HIV infection (Figure 4.73) and secondary neoplastic or infective conditions (Figures 4.74–4.78) are responsible for the seizures in roughly equal proportions. Of the opportunistic infections with a predilection for the central nervous system, the protozoon *Toxoplasma gondii* is the most frequently implicated. Cerebral toxoplasma infection usually presents as meningoencephalitis, although an encephalopathic picture may occur. Seizures are seen in 30% of cases.

The diagnosis is confirmed by positive serology, CSF culture and imaging appearances (Figure 4.79).

Differentiation from the direct effects of HIV infection is important as this is a treatable complication. As it represents a reactivation of pre-existing infection, treatment with sulfadiazine and pyrimethamine has to be lifelong. The condition is fatal if allowed to continue unrecognized; *Toxoplasma* abscesses (Figures 4.80–4.82) were found in 13% of one reported AIDS autopsy series. Encephalitis due to viruses such as cytomegalovirus and varicella zoster can occur in patients with HIV, and may cause a secondary vasculitis (Figure 4.83).

Tuberculosis

Tuberculous meningitis remains rare in developed countries, but is becoming more common with increased immigration and the increase in HIV-associated tuberculosis. The usual presentation is an insidious meningoencephalitis. Other complications include cranial nerve palsies, cerebral infarction and obstructive hydrocephalus. Tuberculomas (Figures 4.85–4.87) account for 5–30% of intracranial mass lesions reported in underdeveloped countries, and may present with focal seizures and signs (Figure 4.87).

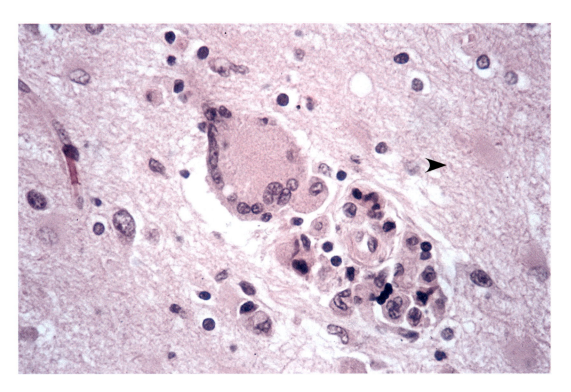

Figure 4.73 HIV encephalitis in AIDS. Histology shows perivascular clusters of virus-infected cells of the monocyte–macrophage series, some of which are multinucleated. There is also evidence of white matter gliosis with gemistocytic astrocytes (arrowed) and demyelination. (H & E)

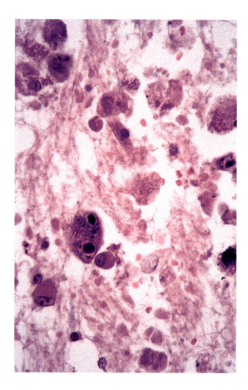

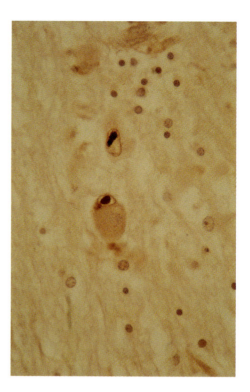

Figure 4.74 Cytomegalovirus encephalitis in AIDS. The presence of conspicuous intranuclear inclusions of viral material in enlarged virus-infected cells characterizes this pathological entity. (H & E)

Figure 4.75 Cytomegalovirus encephalitis in AIDS. Immunohistochemistry for cytomegalovirus antigen confirms its presence within the nuclei of infected cells

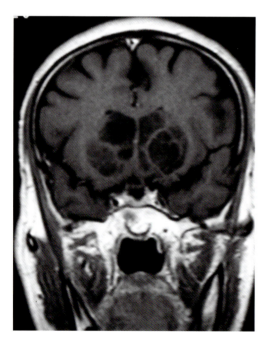

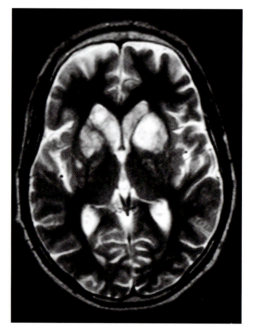

Figure 4.76 Cryptococcal ventriculitis. A 24-year-old man who was known to be HIV positive had a new onset of severe throbbing headache associated with photophobia. Two weeks after the onset, his friends commented that his behavior had altered and he had generally become slower physically. An urgent MRI revealed massive dilatation of the perivascular spaces (Virchow-Robin spaces) in the basal ganglia by cryptococcal infection. Cryptococcus classically spreads through the CSF spaces of the brain causing such dilatation. As they are separated from the brain parenchyma by the blood–brain barrier, these lesions do not show contrast enhancement

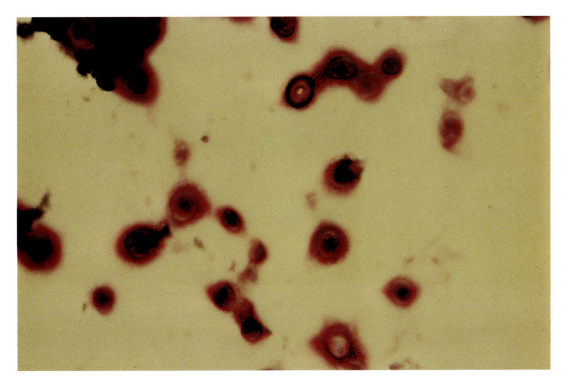

Figure 4.77 Cryptococcal meningitis in AIDS. Cryptococcal meningitis is characterized by a diffuse growth of organisms within the meninges with a minimal associated inflammation. The organisms are readily identifiable by their metachromatic mucoid capsules. (Toluidine blue)

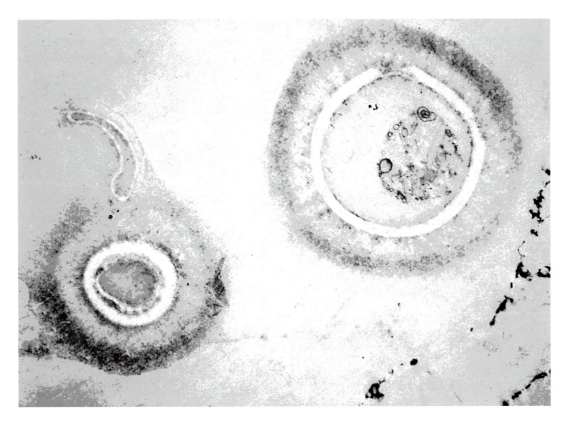

Figure 4.78 Cryptococcal meningitis in AIDS. Electron microscopy showing *Cryptococcus* ultrastructure; the mucoid capsule is readily seen

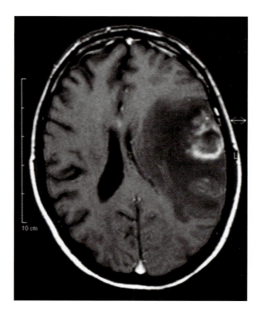

Figure 4.79 Cerebral toxoplasmosis. In a patient with HIV/AIDS who had a single tonic-clonic seizure. MRI scan shows a ring-enhancing lesion at the corticomedullary junction of left parietal lobe with tiny satellite ring enhancing nodules around it. Satellite lesions are seen in toxoplasmosis and in TB; but the site and size of the main lesion and the amount of perifocal edema favor toxoplasmosis. In toxoplasmosis, the extent of contrast enhancement and the amount of edema are directly related to the CD4 count

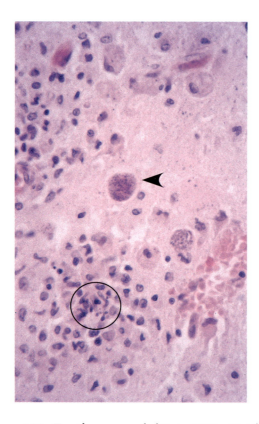

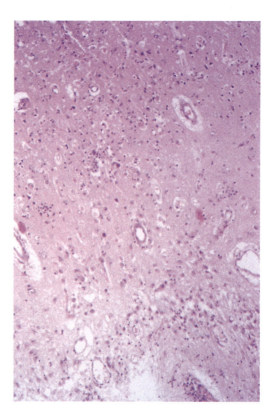

Figure 4.80 *Toxoplasma* encephalitis in AIDS. Histology shows extensive mononuclear inflammation together with the presence of several pseudocysts containing bradyzoites (arrowed); free tachyzoites can also be seen in the tissues (encircled). (H & E)

Figure 4.81 *Toxoplasma* abscess. A 25-year-old male homosexual presented in a comatose state with neck stiffness and seizures. This was treated as bacterial meningitis; death ensued 3 days later. Histology of the cerebral cortex shows focal encephalitic lesions. (H & E; see Figure 4.82)

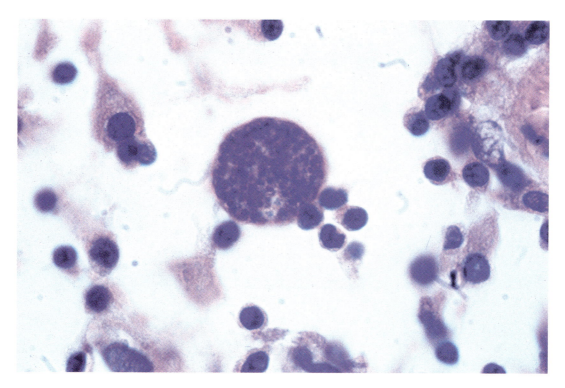

Figure 4.82 *Toxoplasma* abscess. Histology shows a pseudocyst filled with bradyzoites of *Toxoplasma gondii*. (H & E)

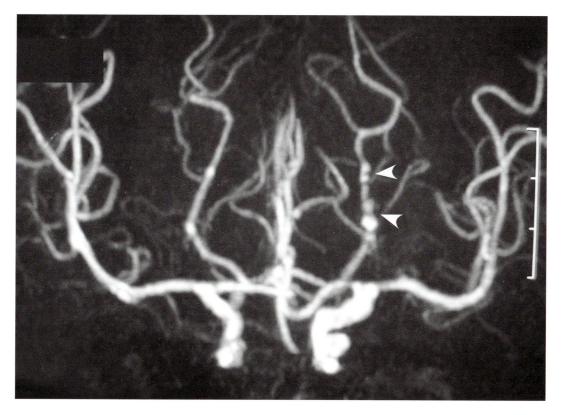

Figure 4.83 Cerebral vasculitis. MR angiography of the circle of Willis in a patient who was HIV positive and presented with an encephalitic illness. The MR angiogram shows 'beading' characteristic of vasculitis, particularly on the left (arrows)

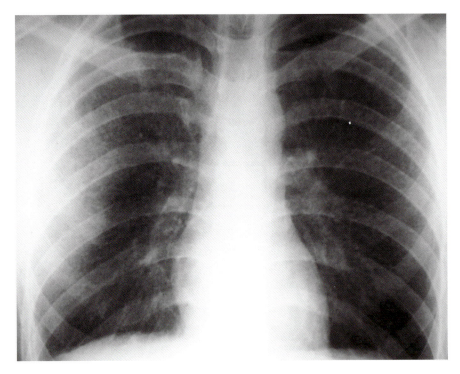

Figure 4.84 Disseminated tuberculosis. A 39-year-old woman from Pakistan presented with a cough and shortness of breath. Chest X-ray at this time showed a small left-sided pleural effusion. A few weeks later she developed a subacute illness characterized by headache, fever and clouding of consciousness. Chest X-ray shows diffuse abnormalities suggestive of military tuberculosis

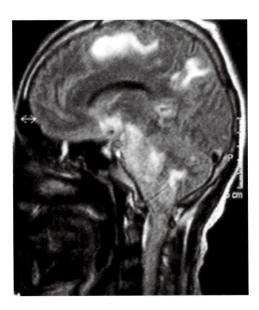

Figure 4.85 Disseminated tuberculosis. MRI FLAIR images (same patient as Figure 4.84) reveal cortical and subcortical high signal changes representing the consequences of extensive vasculitis in a patient with TB. Note the ring-like lesions at the base of the brain extending below foramen magnum (tuberculomas) and the high signal in the spinal meninges (TB meningitis). CSF PCR was positive for TB

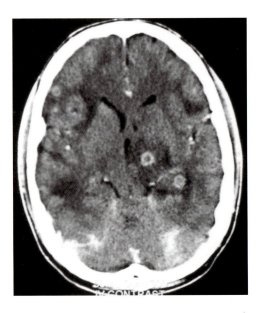

Figure 4.86 Tuberculosis. Post-contrast CT scan demonstrates numerous ring enhancing lesions (tuberculomas) throughout the brain with modest perilesional edema

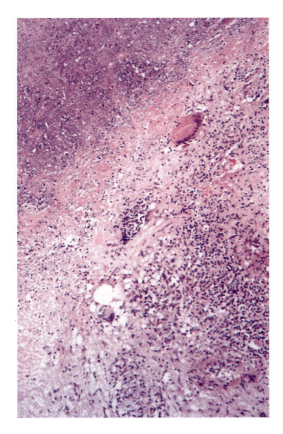

Figure 4.87 Tuberculoma. Histology of the wall of a cerebral tuberculoma shows extensive coagulative necrosis with an adjacent inflammatory reaction, characterized by fibrosis and infiltration by lymphocytes, epithelioid cells and Langerhans' giant cells. (H & E)

Neurosyphilis

Untreated infection with *Treponema pallidum* may affect the central nervous system after a variable (1–30 years) period of latency. Neurosyphilis is classified as tertiary (meningovascular) or quaternary (parenchymatous). The latter involves direct treponemal invasion of the neurons of the cerebrum (general paresis of the insane) or the spinal cord (tabes dorsalis).

General paresis of the insane presents with insidious mental changes and gradually progresses to a profound dementia. Seizures, either focal or generalized, occur in 50% of cases and may be the presenting symptom, whereas focal deficits are a late feature. There is usually a CSF pleocytosis. Specific treponemal tests indicate previous infection and remain positive throughout life, but may be negative with concomitant HIV infections. Non-specific lipoidal tests provide an index of disease activity. The diagnosis requires a high degree of suspicion as early treatment may be effective. However, the prognosis is generally poor with death ensuing within 2–5 years (Figures 4.88 and 4.89).

As with tuberculosis, the incidence of neurosyphilis has increased in recent years, mainly due to HIV disease. In patients with co-existent HIV the disease course is more rapid, and it is more difficult to treat.

Neurocysticercosis

Cysticercosis is the larval stage of infection by the pork tapeworm *Taenia solium*. In both Central and South America, it is the leading cause of epilepsy and other neurological disorders. Other cerebral manifestations include obstructive hydrocephalus, focal deficits and, rarely, subarachnoid hemorrhages. Tonic-clonic seizures are the most common presenting feature. Early treatment with praziquantel abolishes the need for continuing antiepileptic drugs in 70% of cases but, if the lesions calcify (Figure 4.90), a permanent epileptogenic focus may result. The radiographic appearances may be more florid in the untreated patient (Figure 4.91).

Cerebral malaria

Cerebral malaria complicates 2% of infections with falciparum malaria. Children, pregnancy, immunosuppression and cessation of antimalarial prophylaxis increase the risk. A rapidly fatal encephalopathy usually occurs during the second or third week of the illness, but may also be the initial presentation. The appearances on necropsy are characteristic (Figure 4.92).

Subacute sclerosing panencephalitis

This extremely rare (in the 'developed' world) subacute or chronic encephalopathy usually affects children and young adults. It typically presents 6–10 years after primary measles infection and may represent an abnormal immune response. The inexorable course is characterized by dementia, myoclonus, seizures, ataxia, rigidity and death usually, but not invariably, within 1–5 years. The diagnosis is confirmed by the classical EEG (Figure 4.93) and MRI appearances (Figures 4.94), elevated IgG concentrations in the CSF, and raised measles antibody titers in the serum and CSF. The postmortem findings are pathognomonic (Figures 4.95 and 4.96).

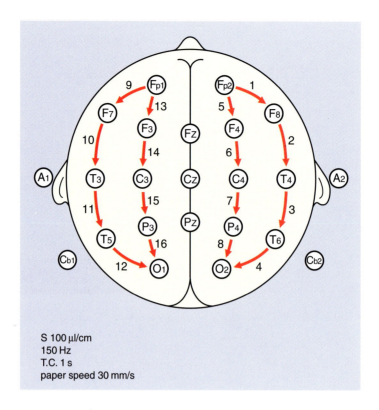

S 100 µl/cm
150 Hz
T.C. 1 s
paper speed 30 mm/s

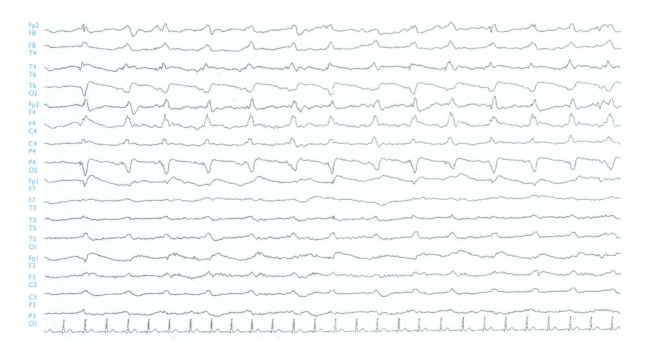

Figure 4.88 Neurosyphilis. A 36-year-old homosexual hairdresser was admitted to hospital on three occasions with secondarily generalized tonic-clonic seizures. On the third occasion, he was transferred to the neurology unit in a confusional state. EEGs revealed complex partial status epilepticus. Despite resolution of his non-convulsive status, his mental state remained abnormal; his work performance had deteriorated during the preceding 10 months. Serological tests in blood and cerebrospinal fluid suggested active neurosyphilis (rapid plasma reagin 1 : 256; TPHA (*Treponema pallidum* hemagglutination) > 1280). After treatment with procaine penicillin and prednisolone, psychometry revealed an IQ of 70 with profound verbal and visual memory deficits. Six months later, he was functioning well at work; at that time, blood and cerebrospinal fluid rapid plasma reagin was negative

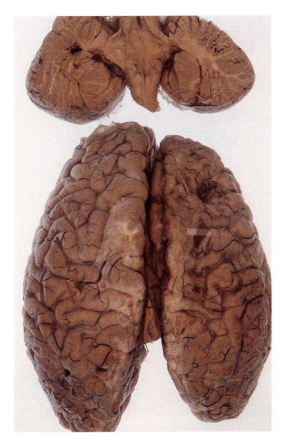

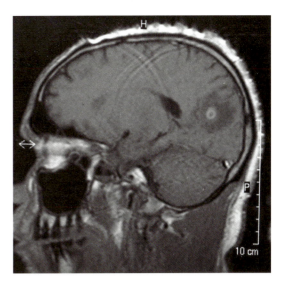

Figure 4.90 Neurocysticercosis. A 35-year-old woman from South Africa presenting acutely in status epilepticus. She was otherwise well but MRI brain scan shows a single lesion in the occipital lobe with some surrounding edema

Figure 4.89 Neurosyphilis. Gross appearances of cerebellum and brain stem (upper), and cerebrum (lower) viewed from above, show changes mainly of meningovascular syphilis with diffuse leptomeningeal thickening. There are multiple areas of cortical infarction particularly in the right hemisphere secondary to endarteritis obliterans of the meningeal arteries; there is right cerebral atrophy

Rasmussen's 'encephalitis' (Rasmussen syndrome)

This rare syndrome usually develops during early to mid-childhood and is characterized by either a gradual or an explosive onset of frequent focal seizures, including epilepsia partialis continua. Progressive hemiplegia and other neurological deficits develop, and death may follow either rapidly or after a period of apparent stabilization. CT or MRI of the affected hemisphere will show progressive atrophy and SPECT or PET will reveal hypometabolism in the affected area and, eventually, in the entire hemisphere.

The etiology of the syndrome is unknown, and previously a low-grade viral infection (particularly

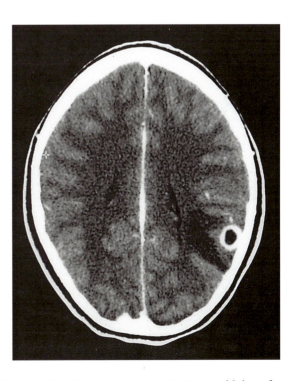

Figure 4.91 Neurocysticercosis. A 7-year-old boy from Pakistan had a 2-month history of recurrent partial seizures, headache and low-grade fever due to infestation with *Taenia solium* (neurocysticercosis). Contrast-enhanced axial CT shows a single ring-enhancing lesion with surrounding edema in the left parietal lobe

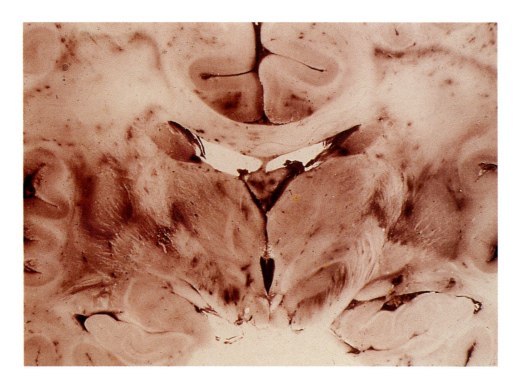

Figure 4.92 Cerebral malaria. Coronal section through the cerebrum at the level of the mammillary bodies shows the typical appearances of fatal malaria due to *Plasmodium falciparum*. There is generalized edema. The numerous petechial hemorrhages, most evident in the white matter of the centrum semiovale and the internal capsules, represent hemorrhage around small vessels occluded by parasitized erythrocytes

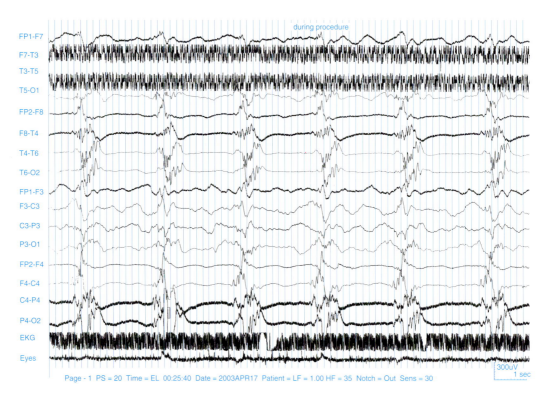

Figure 4.93 EEG of an 11-year-old from Malawi with a 5-month history of myoclonic and tonic-clonic seizures and loss of self-help skills. Admitted with an encephalopathy and a Glasgow Coma Scale score of 8. EEG shows a periodic and burst-suppression pattern with irregular spike and slow-wave activity occurring every 2.5 s, consistent with subacute sclerosing panencephalitis (SSPE) and subsequently confirmed with high titers of measles antibody in the CSF

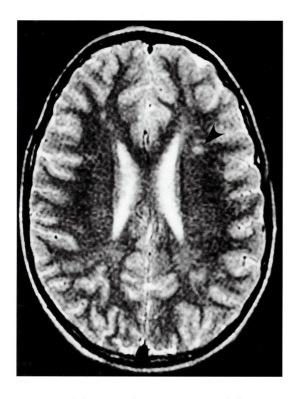

Figure 4.94 Subacute sclerosing panencephalitis. A 13-year-old boy had a history of altered behavior, declining school performance and infrequent generalized tonic-clonic seizures due to subacute sclerosing panencephalitis. T2-weighted MRI shows areas of high signal in the periventricular white matter (arrowed) which are indicative of demyelination

cytomegalovirus) had been implicated. However, in recent years, research has focused on a possible role for antibody-mediated mechanisms and cell-mediated immunity in its pathogenesis. It is likely that there may be a number of different etiologies (Figures 4.97–4.99).

The seizures are resistant to most antiepileptic drugs. The main emphasis of treatment is with immunomodulatory treatment, in particular cortico-steroids, intravenous immunoglobulin, tacrolimus and plasma exchange. Evaluation of the efficacy of such treatments is difficult due to the rarity of the condition. Surgery (usually anatomical hemispherec-tomy or a functional hemispherotomy) is considered to be the treatment of choice in children.

GENETICS OF THE EPILEPSIES

Genetic factors may be implicated in at least 50% of all the epilepsies[1]. A number of inherited disorders are manifested by both epileptic seizures and other paroxysmal disorders (e.g. migraine, stroke-like episodes, paralysis) and several specific epilepsy syndromes have a predominantly genetic basis. Many of these epilepsies and mixed disorders comprising of both epilepsy and other paroxysmal events are now recognized to be caused by abnormalities in ion channel structure and function. Although there have

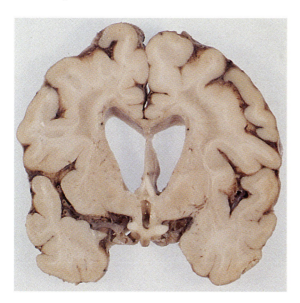

Figure 4.95 Subacute sclerosing panencephalitis. Coronal section of the cerebrum at the level of the optic chiasm shows generalized cerebral atrophy with dilatation of the lateral and third ventricles. The cerebral white matter has been reduced in bulk and shows gray discoloration due to the presence of diffuse gliosis

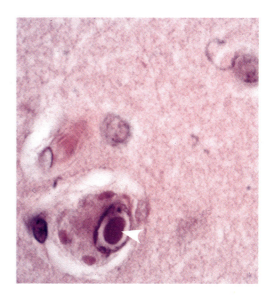

Figure 4.96 Subacute sclerosing panencephalitis. Histology of the cerebral cortex shows several large intranuclear inclusions of measles virus (arrowed). (H & E)

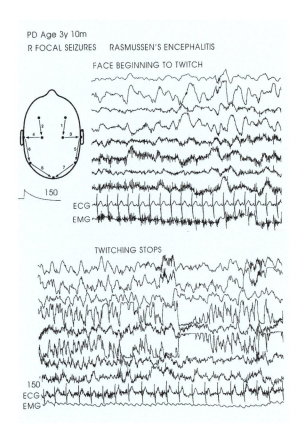

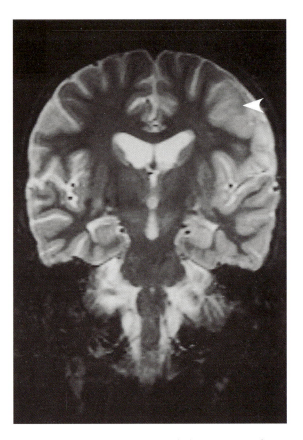

Figure 4.97 Rasmussen's 'encephalitis'. This 4-year-old boy had an 8-month history of increasingly frequent right-sided myoclonic and clonic seizures affecting the face and arm, with secondarily generalized tonic-clonic seizures and episodes of convulsive status epilepticus. EEG shows virtually continuous slow-wave activity in the left frontal region with build-up to a prolonged run of discharges in the frontal and central regions associated with a seizure. The patient developed a progressive right hemiparesis and dysphasia

Figure 4.98 Rasmussen's 'encephalitis'. Coronal MRI (same patient as in Figure 4.97) demonstrates a high-signal and thickened cortex in the left posterior frontal region (arrowed). Brain biopsy of the cortical abnormality confirmed the diagnosis

been – and continue to be – dramatic advances in molecular genetics which have clarified the pathogenesis and inheritance of many of these disorders, these advances have yet to be translated into clear and consistent practical benefits – in terms of specific treatments or specific prognoses. In addition, many of the identified mutational DNA analyses for some of these paroxysmal movement and epileptic disorders are provided by only a limited number of molecular genetic laboratories.

Hereditary disorders and epilepsy

A total of at least 160 Mendelian traits (single-gene defects) are associated with seizures with or without mental retardation. Autosomal recessive traits, which

are often due to enzyme defects, are the most likely to manifest seizures (Table 4.2).

Multifactorial (polygenic) and maternally inherited conditions are also well documented. Examples of the conditions associated with each mode of inheritance are shown in Table 4.3.

The risks of epilepsy occurring in patients with some chromosomal abnormalities are presented in Table 4.4.

Angelman's syndrome

This is a rare disorder that affects children, comprising psychomotor and profound speech and language delay, epilepsy (commonly myoclonic and tonic–atonic seizures) and an abnormal affect characterized by almost continuous smiling and episodes of inappropriate (but 'pleasant' and even infectious) laughter. Because of these latter features and the child's frequent jerky movements, the condition is also

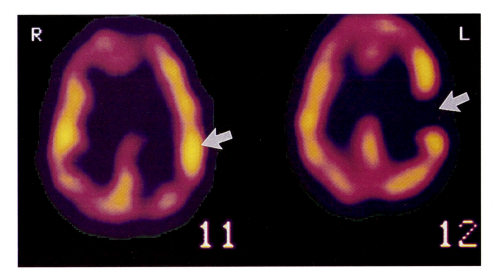

Figure 4.99 Rasmussen's 'encephalitis'. Ictal (left) and interictal (right) technetium-99-labelled HMPAO-SPECT scans (same patient as in Figures 4.97 and 4.98) show a focal area of hyperperfusion and hypoperfusion, respectively, in the left posterior frontal region (arrowed). Intravenous methylprednisolone and immunoglobulins were ineffective. Hemispherectomy was undertaken 4 years and 3 months after diagnosis

Table 4.2 Mendelian traits associated with seizures, with and without mental retardation. From reference 2, with permission

	Total (n)	Seizures and retardation		Seizures only		Total seizures	
		n	%	n	%	n	%
Autosomal dominant	3047	19	0.6	24	0.8	43	1.4
Autosomal recessive	1554	79	5.1	19	1.2	98	6.3
X-linked recessive	1336	15	4.5	4	1.2	19	5.7
Total	4937	113	2.3	47	1.0	160	3.2

sometimes known as the 'happy puppet' syndrome. The EEG may be helpful in establishing the diagnosis (Figure 4.100). The condition has a genetic basis, with approximately 70% of children having an abnormality of chromosome 15.

Rett syndrome

Although Rett syndrome was previously considered to be a relatively rare syndrome affecting only girls, it is clear that there is a far broader phenotype, including that affecting boys. The frequency is currently thought to be approximately 1/5000–10 000. In girls the condition is characterized by developmental regression, acquired microcephaly (usually by 2 years

of age), epilepsy, episodes of hyperventilation (often alternating with apneas) and repetitive stereotypical hand-wringing movements. The epilepsy usually presents after the age of 2 years, but may develop in the first year of life, and usually includes tonic, myoclonic, atonic and prolonged atypical absence seizures. Infantile spasms rarely occur in children with classical Rett syndrome, but typically occur in rarer variants (due to a mutation in the CDKL5/STK9 gene) when the spasms are accompanied by hypsarrhythmia on the EEG (Figure 4.101) that persists well into the second year of life and these patients are usually refractory to treatment. In boys the presentation is often in the neonatal period, or

Table 4.3 Hereditary disorders leading to conditions associated with seizures by mode of inheritance

Mode of inheritance	Condition
Mendelian (symptomatic)	
Autosomal recessive	Unverricht–Lundborg disease
	infantile NCL
	juvenile NCL (Batten disease)
	Lafora body disease
	Northern epilepsy
Autosomal dominant	tuberous sclerosis complex
	neurofibromatosis type I
	Miller–Dieker syndrome
	generalized epilepsy and febrile
	seizures plus (GEFS+)
X-linked	fragile X syndrome
	band heterotopia/lissencephaly
	periventricular nodular
	heterotopia
Mendelian (idiopathic)	
Autosomal dominant	benign familial neonatal
(AD)	convulsions
	benign familial infantile
	convulsions
	AD nocturnal frontal lobe
	epilepsy
	AD partial epilepsies:
	with auditory symptoms
	with speech dyspraxia
	with variable foci
	with temporal lobe epilepsy
Non-Mendelian (idiopathic)	
Complex inheritance	juvenile myoclonic epilepsy
	childhood absence epilepsy
	benign childhood epilepsy with
	centrotemporal spikes
Maternal inheritance	MELAS, MERRF
mitochondrial	
DNA mutations	

NCL, neuronal ceroid lipofuscinosis; MELAS, mitochondrial encephalopathy, lactic acidosis and stroke-like episodes; MERRF, myoclonic epilepsy with ragged red fibers

first few months of life, with frequent, multiple and drug-resistant seizures with death often by the age of 2 or 3 years. Prior to the identification of the common DNA mutation, in the X-linked methyl CpG-binding protein (MECP)2 gene on chromosome Xq28 (found in approximately 75–80% of girls with

Table 4.4 Miscellaneous genetic conditions with epilepsy as a relatively frequent feature

Angelman syndrome – maternally derived deletion on chromosome 15q11-13

Down's syndrome – trisomy 21

Fragile X syndrome – nuclear-derived DNA mutation

Mitochondrial cytopathies
  MERRF (myoclonic epilepsy and ragged red fibers seen on muscle biopsy), caused by a maternally derived DNA point mutation (commonly, amino acid 8344))
  MELAS (mitochondrial encephalopathy, lactic acidosis and stroke-like episodes) in which children may present with or develop focal seizures and epilepsia partialis continua caused by a maternally derived DNA point mutation (commonly, 3234))

Rett syndrome – MECP2 mutation on chromosome Xq28 (plus numerous other mutations within this gene, resulting in variants of the 'classical' Rett syndrome clinical phenotype and mutations in the CDKL5/STK9 gene)

Other chromosomal disorders – trisomy 12 and ring chromosomes 14 and 20

X-linked recessive infantile spasms – mutation on the ARX or homeobox gene

the classic clinical phenotype), EEG was often very helpful in establishing the diagnosis.

Malformations of cortical development

These disorders, also known by such terms as cortical dysgenesis, cortical dysplasia and neuronal migration disorders, differ widely in their clinical presentation, genetic basis and associated pathology. In recent years advances particularly in imaging and genetics have increased our knowledge of the malformations of cortical development (MCD), but this has not generally translated into therapeutic advances[3].

Focal cortical dysplasia (FCD) is an important cause of refractory focal-onset epilepsy usually presenting in childhood. This is the one form (although FCD is unlikely to represent a single entity) of MCD in which advances in imaging may influence outcome, as identification of FCD with high-resolution MRI imaging may lead to surgical treatment. Features on imaging suggestive of FCD are local cortical thickening, blurring of the grey to white matter interface, and increased signal in the underlying white matter (Figures 4.102 and 4.103). Currently the pathogenesis of FCD is unknown, but it is highly probable that there may be a genetic component.

The other most common MCDs that may present with epilepsy are: periventricular heterotopia (nodules of heterotopic grey matter in a periventricular or subcortical location), occurring either sporadically or as an inherited (X-linked dominant) trait (Figure 4.104) polymicrogyria (an excess number of small gyri producing an irregular cortical surface); schizencephaly (a transcortical cleft lined by cortex) (Figures 4.105 and 4.106), subcortical band heterotopia (bands of neurons in the subcortical white matter); and lissencephaly (abnormally smooth brain surface with flat or absent gyri). The current knowledge of the genetics of these conditions are shown in Table 4.5.

GENETICS OF THE EPILEPSIES AND EPILEPSY SYNDROMES

The genetic loci of a number of epilepsies (and epilepsy syndromes) have been mapped to specific chromosomes (Figures 4.107 and 4.108); this number is certain to increase in the next few years. The genetic basis of the idiopathic 'generalized' epilepsies with their characteristic generalized spike-and-wave pattern is well-established – although there is clear overlap – with twin studies indicating that specific seizure types and epilepsy syndromes are inherited within families (Figure 4.109). This knowledge has implications for and may be of use in patient counseling (Figure 4.110). One of the most interesting epilepsy syndromes recently identified (and still being evaluated) is generalized epilepsy and febrile seizures plus (GEFS+) with loci on at least two chromosomes (2q and 19q). In this phenotype, febrile seizures occur, (often well beyond the age of 5 years) in one or more family members, with others in the same family experiencing afebrile generalized seizures (tonic-clonic, absence and myoclonic) occurring throughout childhood and adult life. Children with severe myoclonic epilepsy in infancy (also called Dravet syndrome) have also been reported in this specific syndrome. There is clear evidence that GEFS+ is one of the many – and increasing number of – ion channelopathies, specifically involving one or more sodium channels. It is also becoming increasingly clear that a number of other epilepsies and

epilepsy syndromes are caused by disorders of ion channels and membrane receptors (e.g. a mutation of the neuronal nicotinic acetylcholine receptor gene has been identified in autosomal dominant nocturnal frontal lobe epilepsy).

HEAD INJURIES

The relationship between head injury, acute symptomatic seizures and late post-traumatic epilepsy is well documented. The risk of post-traumatic epilepsy is directly related to the severity of the cerebral insult.

Penetrating head injury

Penetrating head wounds resulting from missile injuries carry a 50% risk of post-traumatic epilepsy. Factors increasing the risk include involvement of the motor-premotor cortex, extent of cerebral tissue loss and, particularly, the development of abscess formation. This type of injury carries the highest relative risk of developing epilepsy of any cerebral insult (Figure 4.111). On 15-year follow-up, more than 50% of patients have active epilepsy.

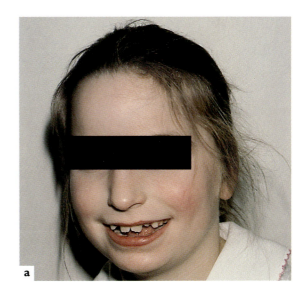

Figure 4.100 Angelman's syndrome. An 8-year-old girl with this syndrome (a) experienced tonic and myoclonic-atonic seizures. EEGs (overleaf) (b) show runs of slow 3-cps waves which are frequently notched (arrowed) and occasionally associated with true spikes

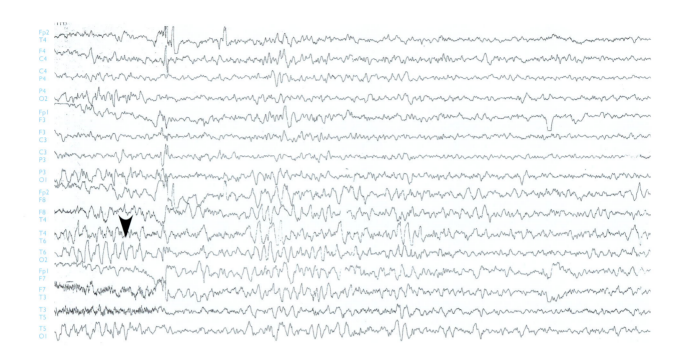

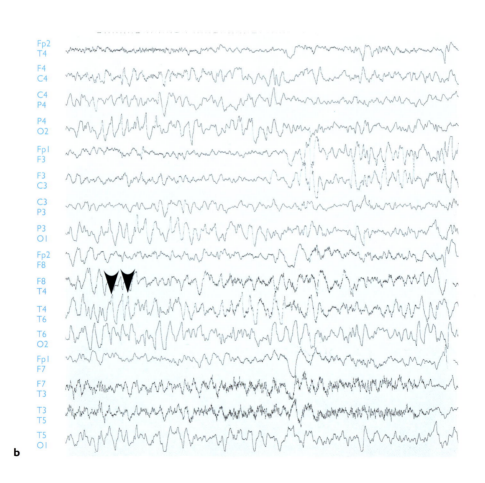

Figure 4.100 *continued*

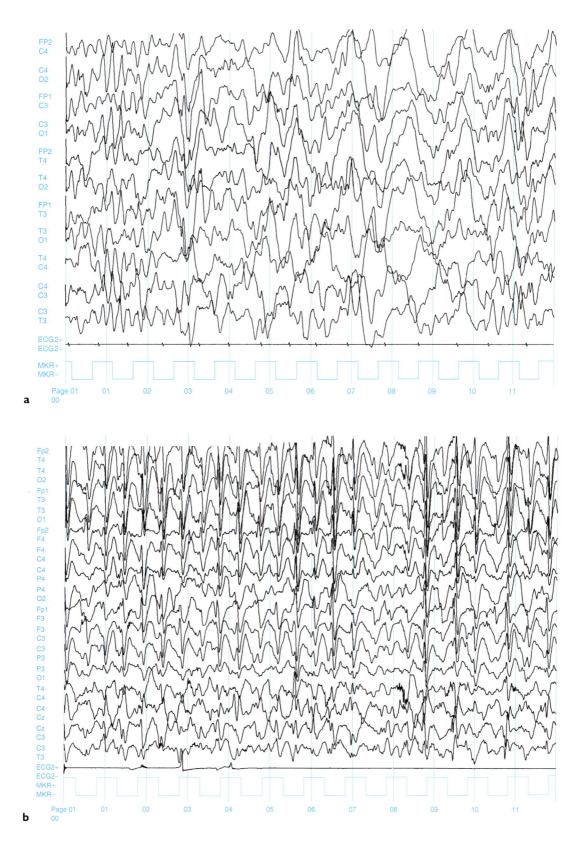

Figure 4.101 (a) Sleeping EEG of a 3½-year-old girl with MECP2-confirmed Rett syndrome showing a grossly abnormal background consistent with an almost hypsarrhythmic pattern. (b) Waking EEG of the same girl (but aged 6 years) with frequent episodes of atypical absence status showing regular and continuous slow (2–2.5 Hz) spike and slow-wave activity. During these periods which lasted from between 30 s and 3 min and recurring every 2–5 min, she would simply stare ahead with no head or eye deviation or automatisms and with no obvious change in her respiratory pattern. *Continued*

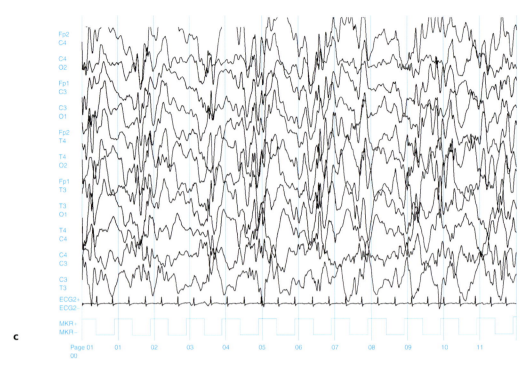

c

Figure 4.101 *continued.* (c) EEG of a 23-month-old girl with Rett syndrome and with a mutation of the CDKL5 gene showing persistent hypsarrhythmia; infantile spasms had developed from 3 months of age and had been resistant to all antiepileptic drugs but had shown some partial response to pyridoxal phosphate

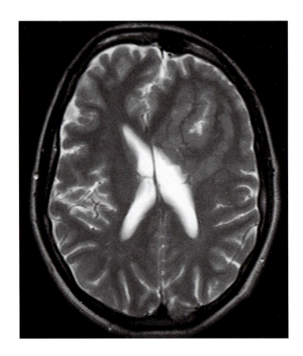

Figure 4.102 Focal cortical dysplasia. A 28-year-old woman presented with nocturnal seizures, which were refractory to antiepileptic drug treatment. The seizures consist of tingling followed by weakness in the right arm, which then evolves into a dystonic posture and then a secondarily generalized tonic-clonic seizure. Her early development was normal. MRI scan showed an extensive area of focal cortical dysplasia in the left hemisphere

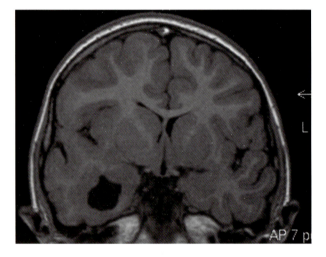

Figure 4.103 Focal cortical dyslasia. A 6-year-old boy with a 4-year history of complex partial seizures and rare and waking, secondarily generalized tonic-clonic seizures. Coronal, T1-weighted image shows focal cortical dysplasia in the right temporal lobe. The affected cerebral cortex is thickened and poorly differentiated from the underlying white matter; there is also dilatation of the temporal horn of the right lateral ventricle. The left temporal lobe appears normal and in particular shows a normal cortical thickness and normal gray–white matter differentiation

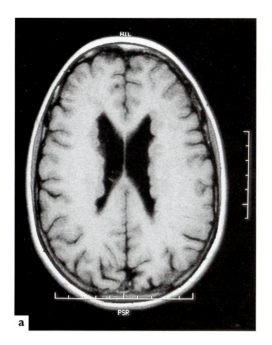
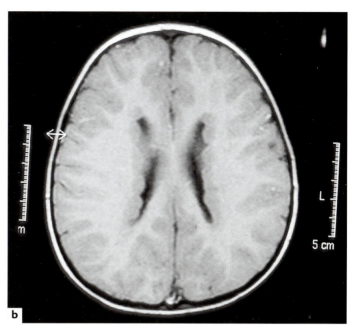

Figure 4.104 Familial (X-linked) bilateral periventricular nodular heterotopia. Mother (a) and daughter (b) who presented at 25 and 3 years of age, respectively, with generalized tonic-clonic seizures which were controlled with sodium valproate (mother) and carbamazepine (daughter). Axial T1-weighted MRI shows multiple nodular masses lining the lateral ventricles that are isodense with cortical gray matter (thereby indicating that the nodules represent heterotopic gray matter)

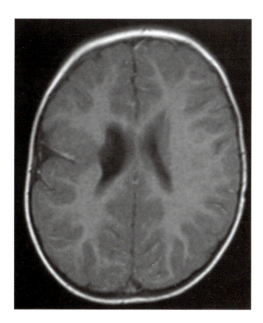

Figure 4.105 Unilateral closed lip schizencephaly. A 23-year-old man presenting with nocturnal partial and secondarily generalized tonic-clonic seizures. Axial T1-weighted MRI shows right closed lip schizencephaly. Bulky gray matter extends from the cortex to the ventricular surface of the dilated right lateral ventricle. A large dimple in the ventricular wall indicates the opening of the cleft into the lateral ventricle. The entire cortex of the right hemisphere (particularly frontally) is bulky and thickened, suggesting pachygyria

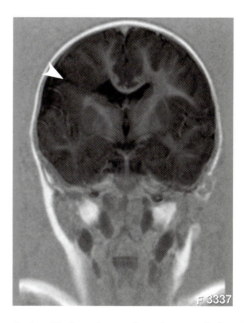

Figure 4.106 Unilateral open lip schizencephaly. A 30-year-old man with refractory partial (focal) seizures and a mild left hemiparesis. Coronal MRI demonstrates right open lip schizencephaly, a dilated frontal horn of the right lateral ventricle and thickened gray matter extending from the cortex to the ventricular surface. The cleft is very narrow (arrow)

Table 4.5 The genetics of the malformations of cortical development

Malformation	Gene	Clinical features
Focal cortical dysplasia	unknown	often presents in first decade; frequently drug-refractory focal-onset epilepsy; may cause focal motor status or epilepsia partialis continua; may present with neonatal encephalopathy
Periventricular heterotopia	FLNA – Xq28 encodes filamin A, a protein essential for neuronal migration; other genes are also likely to be involved: recessive inheritance and locus on chromosome 5 described	mutations cause epilepsy (which may be refractory to treatment) in females presenting in or after the second decade, usually with normal intellect; may be associated with hippocampal sclerosis (see Figure 6.49) but surgery unsuccessful; can rarely occur in males
Polymicrogyria and schizencephaly	various linkages to different chromosomal regions reported MECP2 – found in male patient with bilateral perisylvian polymicrogyria and neonatal encephalopathy PAX6 – homeobox gene – mutations can cause unilateral polymicrogyria	can be unilateral or bilateral; may present with developmental delay or congenital hemiparesis; bilateral perisylvian polymicrogyria – pseudobulbar palsy, spastic quadriplegia, learning disability and epilepsy
Subcortical band heterotopia lissencephaly	DCX – X chromosome encodes doublecortin, a protein involved in neuronal migration LIS1 – 17p13.3	mutations can cause sporadic lissencephaly in males, subcortical band heterotopia in females, or a mixture within a single kindred; deletions or point mutations can cause isolated lissencephaly; heterozygous deletions lead to Miller-Dieker syndrome with severe lissencephaly, craniofacial defects and early death

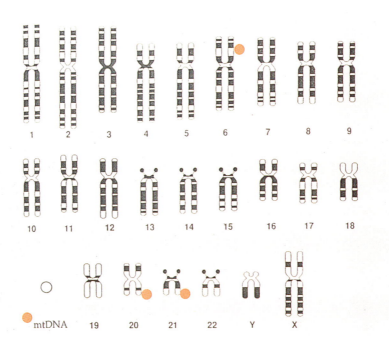

Figure 4.107 Human karyotype. The orange spots indicate the first three chromosomes which are relevant to epilepsy syndromes

Mendelian epilepsy gene map (autosomal)		
Dominantly inherited conditions		
Epilepsy	*Gene locus*	*Gene product*
Autosomal dominant nocturnal frontal lobe epilepsy	20q	CHRNA4
Benign neonatal familial convulsions	20q	?CHRNA4
Generalized epilepsy and febrile seizures plus (GEFS+)	2q and 19q	
Huntington's disease	4p16	huntingtin
Neurofibromatosis 1	17q 11.2	neurofibromin
Partial epilepsies	10q 2.3	
Tuberous sclerosis complex 1	9q 3.4	hamartin
Tuberous sclerosis complex 2	6p 13	tuberin
Recessively inherited conditions		
Epilepsy	*Gene locus*	*Gene product*
Early infantile neuronal ceroid lipofuscinosis	1q	palmitoyl protein thioesterase
Late infantile neuronal ceroid lipofuscinosis	11p 1.5	palmitoyl protein thioesterase
Juvenile neuronal ceroid lipofuscinosis	16p	
Lafora body disease	6q	
Miller-Dieker syndrome	17p	
Unverricht–Lundborg disease	21q 22	cystatin B
Undetermined inheritance		
Epilepsy	*Gene locus*	*Gene product*
Juvenile myoclonic epilepsy	6p; 15q	

Figure 4.108 Mendelian epilepsy gene map. These 14 conditions have been linked to specific chromosomes. In most instances, the gene product has been identified

Blunt trauma

The risks of early seizures (within 1 week of the head injury) and post-traumatic epilepsy in an unselected population of patients with blunt head trauma (Table 4.6) are clearly related to the severity of the insult (Table 4.7). The relative risk of such patients developing epilepsy falls over time (12.7 at 1 year, 4.4 at 1–5 years and 1.4 after 5 years). Table 4.8 shows the definitions of mild, moderate and severe head injury.

In a selected population referred to a neurological center, 5% of survivors developed post-traumatic epilepsy. Significant risk factors (Table 4.9) included early seizures, depressed skull fracture with dural laceration (Figure 4.112) and intracranial hematoma (Figures 4.113–4.115).

On 15-year follow-up, 50% of patients will be in a 5-year remission of seizures, whereas 25% will experience more than six seizures per year. Despite the ability to predict which patients have a high risk of developing post-traumatic epilepsy, prospective controlled studies have failed to demonstrate any benefit of prophylactic antiepileptic agents[6].

Post-traumatic epilepsy is often resistant to antiepileptic medication.

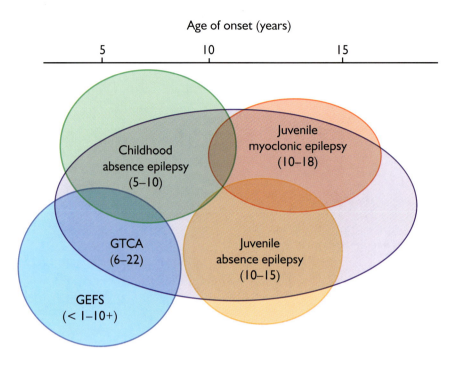

Figure 4.109 Age of onset and overlap of the different epilepsy syndromes within the category of primary generalized epilepsy. (GEFS+, generalized epilepsy with febrile seizures 'plus'; the age of onset of patients with GEFS+ may be considerably older than shown in the figure). Modified from reference 4

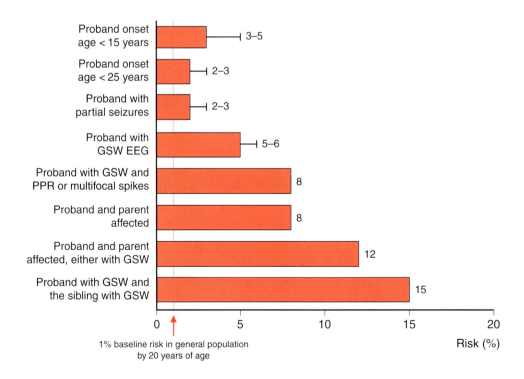

Figure 4.110 Sibling risk for epilepsy. GSW, generalized spike and wave; PPR, photoparoxysmal response. With permission from reference 5

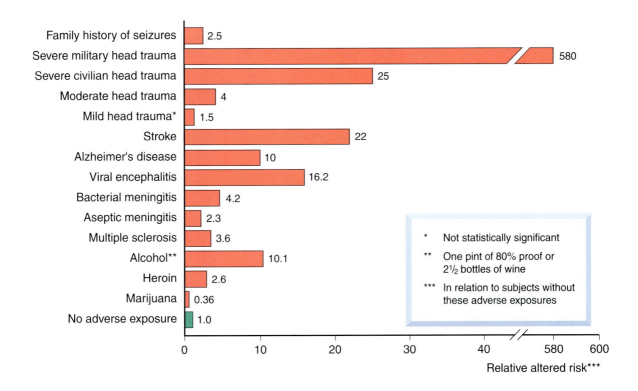

Figure 4.111 Risk of epilepsy associated with various cerebral insults

Table 4.6 Risk of early seizures following blunt head trauma

	Adults (%)	Children (%)
Overall	1.8	2.8
Severe head injury	10.3	30.5

Table 4.7 Risk of late epilepsy following blunt head trauma according to severity of injury

Severity	1 year (%)	5 years (%)
Severe	7.1	11.5
Moderate	0.7	1.6
Mild	0.1	0.6

CEREBRAL TUMORS

Primary intracranial neoplasms are rare. It is now generally accepted that they arise *de novo* as a result of neoplastic transformation of elements in adults. Environmental factors are probably of etiological

Table 4.8 Definitions of mild, moderate and severe head injury

Degree	Definition
Severe	brain contusion, intracerebral or intracranial hematoma, or 24 h of unconsciousness or amnesia; Glasgow Coma Scale (GCS) score of ≤8
Moderate	skull fracture, or 30 min–24 h of unconsciousness or post-traumatic amnesia; GCS score of 9–12
Mild	Briefer periods of unconsciousness or amnesia; GCS score of ≥13

Table 4.9 Risk factors for post-traumatic epilepsy

Risk factor	Incidence (%)
Intracranial hematoma	33
Early seizures	25
Depressed skull fracture	24*

*The risk is doubled if post-traumatic amnesia lasts >24 h

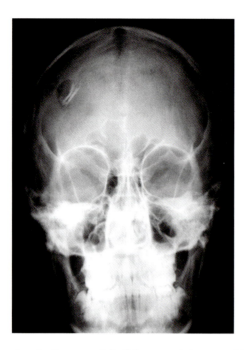

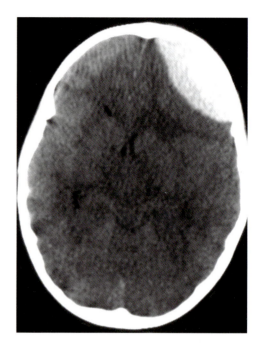

Figure 4.112 Depressed skull fracture. A 21-year-old man was struck on the head with a hammer and was admitted to hospital in generalized convulsive status. Plain skull X-ray shows a depressed fracture in the left parietal region close to the midline. The fracture is comminuted and two large fragments are depressed well into the brain

Figure 4.113 Left frontal extradural hematoma. A 38-year-old woman pedestrian injured in a road traffic accident sustained a closed head injury when her head hit the road; a 'convulsion' occurred within minutes of the injury. Axial CT shows a characteristic left frontal extradural hematoma with obliteration of the frontal horn of the left lateral ventricle, midline shift and mild swelling of the entire left hemisphere. Surgical evacuation of the hematoma was undertaken; the patient had not experienced any epileptic seizures at the time of her final 2-year follow-up

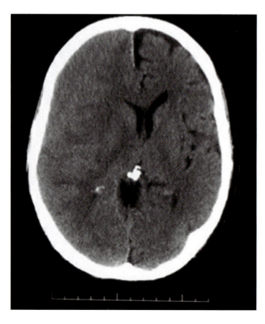

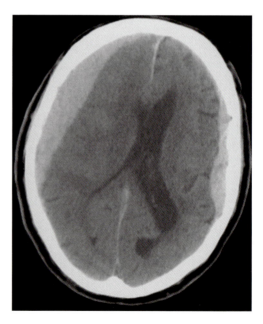

Figure 4.114 Subdural hematoma. CT scan shows a right subdural hematoma that is isodense to brain tissue, indicating that this is 1–3 weeks after the bleed

Figure 4.115 Chronic subdural hematoma. CT scan shows bilateral chronic subdural hematomas. The blood is hypodense to brain tissue over 3 weeks from the bleed

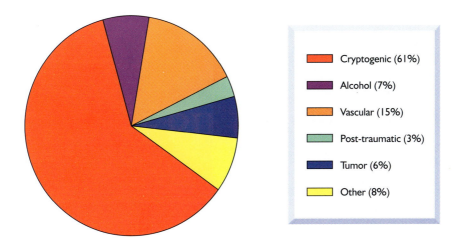

Figure 4.116 National General Practice Study of Epilepsy: etiology of newly diagnosed epilepsy

importance but, apart from radiation, no specific factor has been implicated.

Seizures are a common presentation of primary cerebral tumors, but tumors are a relatively rare cause of epilepsy especially in children. In the National General Practice Study of Epilepsy, a tumor was identified in 6% of all new cases (Figure 4.116), but accounted for 19% of cases involving patients aged 40–59 years. The diagnosis should be suspected in patients with late-onset partial epilepsy, especially if there are focal signs, focal slow waves on the EEG, or a poor initial response to treatment.

Tumors are a relatively rare cause of epilepsy in children, being responsible for between 1 and 2% of all seizure types, and 3 and 5% of focal or partial seizures. This reflects the usual infratentorial (posterior fossa or brainstem) siting of pediatric tumors, particularly in children under 6 years of age. However, in children with brain tumors, 10–20% may have an initial presentation with focal or secondarily generalized tonic-clonic seizures. These tumors are usually relatively benign and are primitive neuro-ectodermal tumors (PNETs), dysembryoblastic neuroepithelial tumors (DNETs) (Figure 4.117), or astrocytomas and less commonly, oligodendrogliomas or meningiomas. Rarely, brain tumors may present soon after birth and may be relatively large and aggressive (Figure 4.118). MRI is far superior to CT in demonstrating a PNET, DNET, or oligodendroglioma, particularly if these are sited in the temporal lobe.

Presentation with epilepsy is a favorable prognostic factor (Figure 4.119) in patients with tumors, and

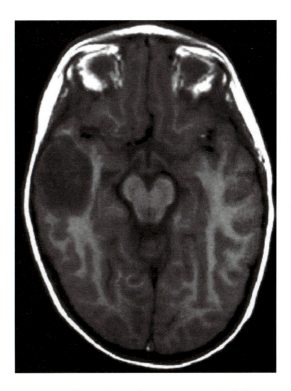

Figure 4.117 Dysembryoplastic neuroepithelial tumor (DNET). A 20-year-old man presented with events characterized by a sensation in his epigastrium rising to his head followed by loss of awareness and orofacial automatisms. He had never experienced any tonic-clonic seizures, but his complex partial seizures were resistant to antiepileptic medication. He had no focal sensorimotor deficit and had an equivocal (inconsistent) defect in his left superior quadrantic visual field. Axial, T1-weighted MRI demonstrates a large and well-circumscribed lesion of near-uniform density in the right temporal lobe with minimal mass (compressive) effect. The patient became seizure-free following a right temporal lobectomy

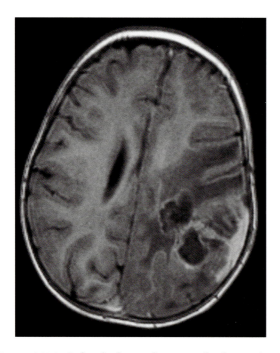

Figure 4.118 Infantile desmoplastic ganglioglioma. A 10-month-old infant presented with a 2-week history of six focal motor seizures affecting her right arm and face, each episode was followed by weakness lasting a number of hours. She had become very irritable and had stopped feeding 24 hours prior to admission. Axial MRI shows a large peripheral tumor in the left cerebral hemisphere with fluid-filled cystic components and surrounded by marked edema of the white matter. The differential diagnosis included a primitive neuroectodermal tumor (PNET); open biopsy confirmed an infantile desmoplastic ganglioglioma

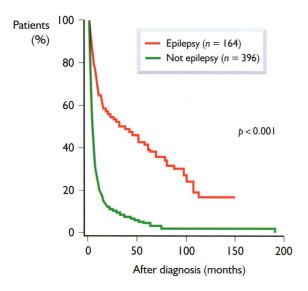

Figure 4.119 Influence of presentation with epilepsy on survival experience of patients with cerebral tumors

may be the only manifestation for years, reflecting a relatively benign underlying pathology. Indeed, although low-grade astrocytomas and oligodendrogliomas are complicated by epilepsy in 60–90% of cases, malignant gliomas usually present with progressive focal deficits.

A number of other clinical and imaging features are useful as prognostic indicators (Table 4.10). Although aggressive management improves survival in cases with highly malignant tumors, such an approach is not of proven value in cases of slow-growing lesions presenting with epilepsy (Table 4.11).

Tumor-associated epilepsy is particularly resistant to antiepileptic drugs and the outcome of surgery depends on the resectability of the lesion.

Some intracranial tumors may be treated with radiotherapy, which can in itself carry complications. Delayed cerebral radiation necrosis (Figure 4.120) is the best described late complication of cerebral radiation, and can cause headache, personality change, focal deficits and seizures. These symptoms can develop insidiously, from 4 months to a number of years following treatment.

Glioblastoma multiforme

This highly malignant astrocytic tumor is the most common glioma affecting the cerebral hemispheres in adults. Seizures occur in 30–40% of patients, but focal signs and enhancing lesions on imaging scanning (Figure 4.121) are usually found at presentation. These lesions are large and frequently involve both hemispheres (Figure 4.122). The histological appearances are characteristic (Figure 4.123).

Low-grade astrocytoma

These relatively benign tumors often cause refractory partial epilepsy in neurologically intact patients. The initial imaging scan usually shows a non-enhancing low-density lesion (Figure 4.124). With time, neurological deficits develop and the imaging appearances indicate increased tumor activity.

These slow-growing lesions are diffusely infiltrative (Figure 4.125) and rarely amenable to complete surgical excision. The histological appearances are typical (Figure 4.126).

Oligodendroglioma

These tumors account for less than 10% of all gliomas and are seen more frequently in male

Table 4.10 Relative risk (RR) of mortality associated with different variables (whole study population) using Cox's stepwise proportional hazards model

	Beta	p Value	RR (95% CI)
Age	0.0218	< 0.0001	
First symptom of epilepsy	–0.7815	< 0.0001	0.46 (0.34, 0.61)
Deep X-ray therapy	–0.7849	< 0.0001	0.46 (0.36, 0.57)
Non-resective surgery	0.5666	< 0.0001	1.76 (1.43, 2.17)
Focal signs	0.4483	0.0001	1.56 (1.24, 1.97)
Enhancement on CT	0.3999	0.0018	1.49 (1.16, 1.92)
Cyst on CT	–0.2822	0.0124	0.75 (0.60, 0.94)

Table 4.11 Relative risk (RR) of mortality associated with different variables (first symptom of epilepsy) using Cox's stepwise proportional hazards model

	Beta	p Value	RR (95% CI)
Focal signs	1.0972	< 0.0001	3.0 (1.86, 4.81)
Age	0.0425	< 0.0001	
Enhancement on CT	1.0044	0.0001	2.73 (1.65, 3.79)
Non-resective surgery	0.8790	0.0002	2.45 (1.52, 3.82)
Gender	0.4571	0.0474	1.58 (1.01, 2.56)

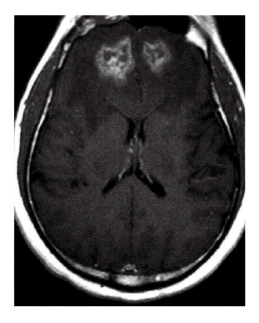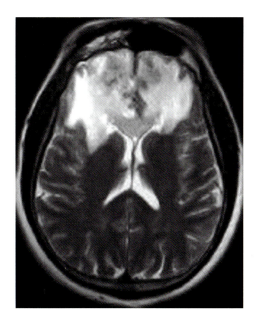

Figure 4.120 Radiation necrosis. A 50-year-old man developed drug-resistant nocturnal complex partial and tonic-clonic seizures 4 years following radiotherapy for a glioma. T2-weighted MRI image (on the right) shows extensive high signal throughout both frontal lobes in a bat's wing distribution. Post-contrast T1-weighted (on left) image shows deep circular enhancement. These changes were proven by biopsy to represent radiation necrosis. Distinction from tumor recurrence can be impossible on standard imaging

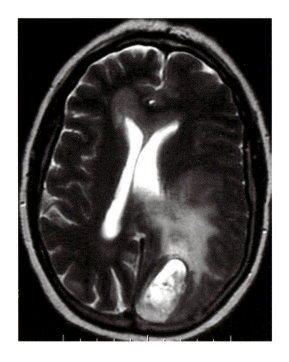

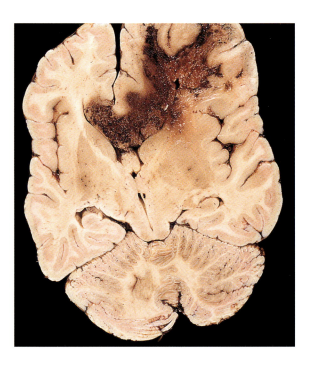

Figure 4.121 Glioblastoma multiforme. A 51-year-old man gave a 2-month history of headache and visual disturbance. He then experienced a single witnessed generalized tonic-clonic seizure. Examination revealed a right homonymous hemianopia and papilledema. MRI shows an irregular mass in the left occipital region with surrounding edema

Figure 4.122 Glioblastoma multiforme. Horizontal section of the brain shows a large glioblastoma involving much of the right frontal lobe and extending into the opposite hemisphere through the corpus callosum. Much of the tumor has undergone hemorrhagic necrosis, but a rim of viable tumor is identifiable diffusely infiltrating the structures of the right frontal pole

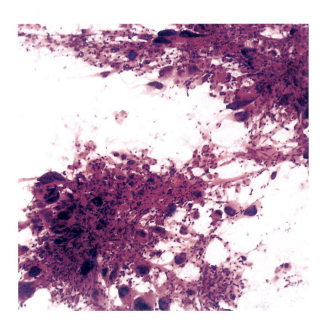

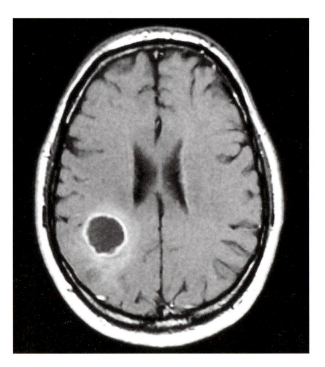

Figure 4.123 Glioblastoma multiforme. Smear preparation of a glioblastoma reveals the characteristic pleomorphic population of poorly differentiated astrocytes. (H & E)

Figure 4.124 Astrocytoma. Post-contrast axial T1-weighted MRI demonstrates ring enhancement within the capsule of an astrocytoma with central necrosis

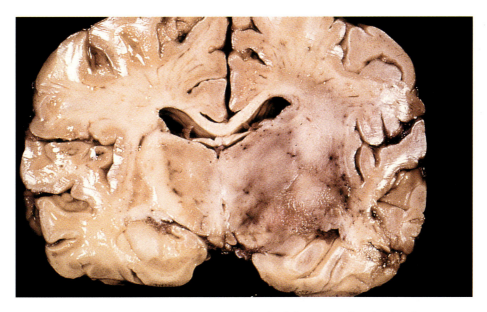

Figure 4.125 Low-grade astrocytoma. Coronal section at the level of the mammillary bodies shows an extensive, diffusely infiltrating, neoplasm in the right hemisphere effacing the basal ganglia, thalamus and surrounding structures

patients. Calcification (Figure 4.127) occurs in more than 50% of lesions, probably as a reflection of their slow growth rate, and is also visible on CT scanning (Figure 4.128).

Surgery and radiotherapy are of no proven benefit in the management of these patients. However, these lesions may sometimes regress with chemotherapy using the nitrogen mustards (*N,N*-

bis(2-chloroethyl)-*N*-nitrosourea and *N*-(2-chloro-ethyl)-*N'*-cyclohexyl-*N*-nitrosourea).

Meningioma

These benign tumors usually arise from arachnoid cells, but may be derived from dural fibroblasts. They comprise 15% of intracranial tumors and are more commonly seen in women. Peak onset is in the

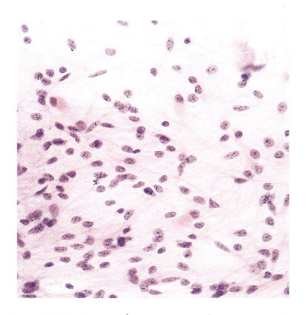

Figure 4.126 Low-grade astrocytoma. Smear preparation reveals a diffuse growth of well-differentiated astrocytes often forming conspicuous fibrillary processes. (H & E)

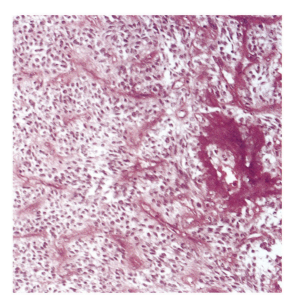

Figure 4.127 Oligodendroglioma. Histology typically shows a diffuse growth of small rounded cells with an intricate capillary network and foci of calcification. (H & E)

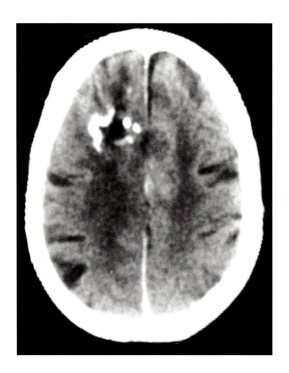 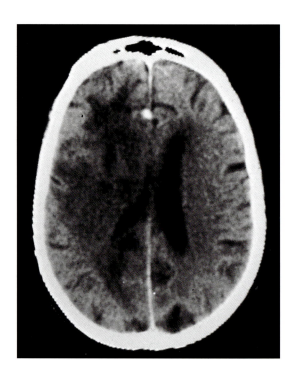

Figure 4.128 Oligodendroglioma. A woman presented with partial seizures in her mid-forties. Epilepsy was the only manifestation for 10 years but, thereafter, she deteriorated progressively with increasing fit frequency, progressive cognitive decline and a right hemiparesis. CTs show a zone of calcification in the left frontal region, with surrounding low density and mass effect

seventh decade, but they may occur earlier in patients with a history of deep X-ray therapy to the scalp or cranium.

The sylvian regions are a site of predilection, and presentation with focal seizures is common. Erosion of the overlying bone is often seen on imaging scanning (Figures 4.129 and 4.130). Accessible surface lesions should be excised (Figure 4.131), but recurrence is possible if excision is not complete. Benign histological features are typical (Figure 4.132).

Developmental cysts

Benign developmental cysts such as arachnoid (of mesenchymal origin) or neuroepithelial (of ependymal origin) cysts can occur throughout the neuroaxis, but when present intracranially may present with epilepsy. It is uncertain as to whether seizures are caused by the cyst or secondary to associated abnormalities such as callosal dysgenesis or cortical dysplasia around the cyst. Symptoms depend on their location, and they are often asymptomatic and discovered incidentally, however, they may cause increased intracranial pressure due to accumulation of CSF-like fluid. Supratentorial arachnoid cysts are

most commonly found in the region of the sylvian fissure and anterior temporal lobe (Figure 4.133), whereas neuroepithelial and other congenital (developmental) cysts are usually near the midline and often close to the ventricular system (Figure 4.134 and 4.135).

Cerebral secondaries

In adults, metastatic carcinoma is much more common than primary intracranial tumors. The most common primary sites, in order of frequency, are the lung, breast, skin (melanoma), colon and kidney. The lung and breast alone account for 50% of cerebral metastases. On imaging, lesions usually appear to be solid and well circumscribed with marked local edema (Figures 4.136–4.138). Metastases are frequently multiple. Cerebral secondaries occur rarely in children.

Primary cerebral lymphoma

This tumor corresponds to the histiocytic type of malignant lymphoma in the Rappaport classification system. It is rare, but the incidence is increasing. Patients with AIDS and long-term immuno-

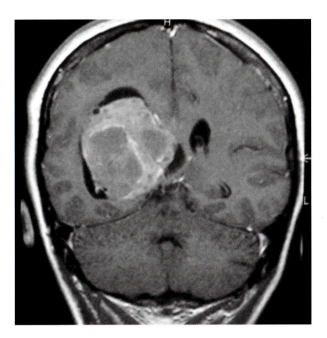

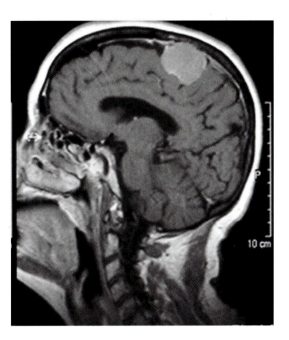

Figure 4.129 Meningioma. A woman presented with brief episodes of a rising epigastric sensation and deja vu. MRI shows a large contrast enhancing mass filling the right lateral ventricle which proved to be a meningioma at surgery. This had obviously been growing for some time yet the patient's only complaints were of these temporal lobe phenomena

Figure 4.130 Meningioma. A post-contrast T1-weighted sagittal MR shows a typical meningioma. Note avid and homogeneous enhancement, clear tumor outline and typical 'dural tail' anterior and posterior to mass

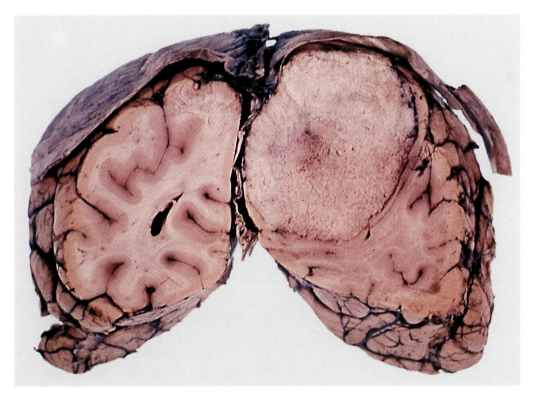

Figure 4.131 Meningioma. Coronal section of cerebrum in parieto-occipital region shows a typically well demarcated meningioma attached to, but not invading, the underlying brain

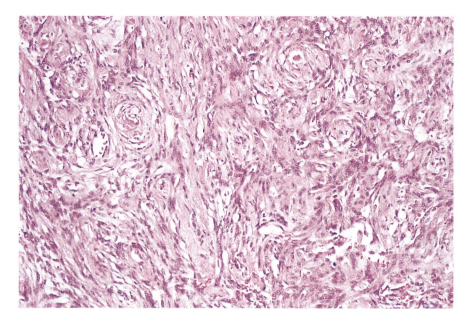

Figure 4.132 Meningioma. Histology consists of well-differentiated meningothelial (arachnoidal) cells growing in sheets and whorls. (H & E)

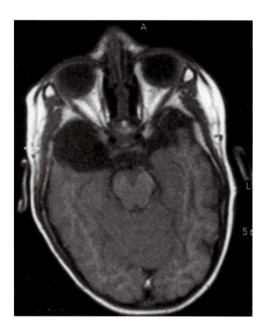

Figure 4.133 Arachnoid cysts (bitemporal; right > left). An almost 3-year-old child with congenital microcephaly and global developmental delay who developed frequent myoclonic seizures from 6 months of age; the EEG demonstrated generalized polyspike and slow wave activity. Axial, T1-weighted MRI demonstrates a large fluid-filled cyst in the right middle cranial fossa and a similar though much smaller cyst in the left middle cranial fossa. The right cyst is consistent with an arachnoid cyst which appears to be exerting some pressure on the adjacent right temporal lobe, although it may have no relevance to the child's epilepsy (co-incidentally, the myelination pattern is somewhat delayed in this child)

suppression, especially renal-transplant patients, are at particular risk. In patients who are not immuno-suppressed, there is some evidence that the Epstein–Barr virus may be causative.

The clinical presentation is similar to that of malignant gliomas but, on imaging, the appearances may be strikingly different (Figure 4.139).

There may be dramatic clinical and radiological improvement after treatment with steroids, but this positive response is only temporary with a median survival of 24 months. Postmortem examination reveals the malignant features of these lesions (Figures 4.140 and 4.141).

CEREBROVASCULAR DISEASE

In the National General Practice Study of Epilepsy[7], a large community-based study, there was evidence of cerebrovascular disease in 15% of patients with newly diagnosed epilepsy. This is the most common cause of epilepsy in the elderly, accounting for up to one-third of cases.

Hemorrhagic strokes carry a much greater risk of epilepsy than do ischemic events (Figure 4.142). The 1-year risk after a subarachnoid hemorrhage is 20%, but this increases after a middle cerebral artery aneurysm has been clipped (see below). The incidence is even greater in patients with arteriovenous

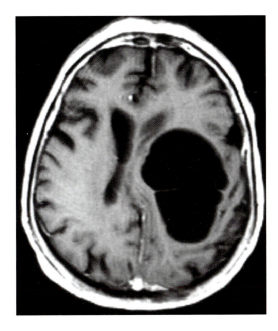

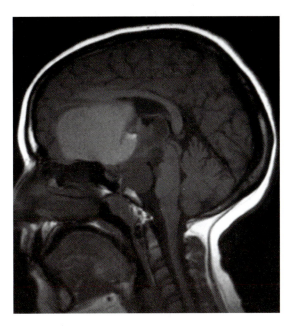

Figure 4.134 Neuroepithelial cyst. A 25-year-old man with a 7-month history of sensory seizures affecting his right face and arm; he had never experienced any tonic-clonic seizures. He had a short history of nocturnal headaches but had no demonstrable neurological deficit. Axial, T1-weighted MRI shows a very large arachnoid cyst with a thin septum within the left cerebral hemisphere and exerting obvious mass effect. Separation of the septum and shunting of the cyst resulted in resolution of his headache and cessation of the seizures

Figure 4.135 Craniopharyngioma. A 14-year-old boy (a refugee from Bosnia) with a 5-year history of infrequent and brief 'absences' (subsequently diagnosed as partial seizures) and two generalized tonic-clonic seizures. On examination he was of short stature and had an asymmetric, bitemporal visual field defect. Parasagittal, T1-weighted MRI demonstrates a very large suprasellar cystic mass, grossly enlarged pituitary and posterior displacement and compression of the pons. Following decompression the child has developed more obvious (though brief and infrequent) complex partial seizures

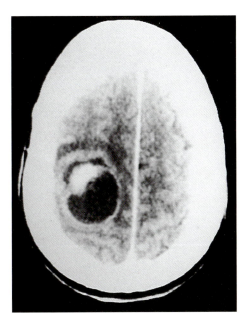

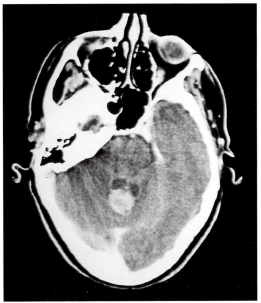

Figure 4.136 Cerebral secondaries. A 60-year-old man had undergone a left pneumonectomy for bronchial carcinoma at the age of 54. He presented with truncal ataxia, focal motor seizures and progressive left-arm weakness. CTs show an enhancing area within the vermis causing slight distortion of the fourth ventricle. There is also an area of ring-shaped enhancement in the right parietal region with a cystic component

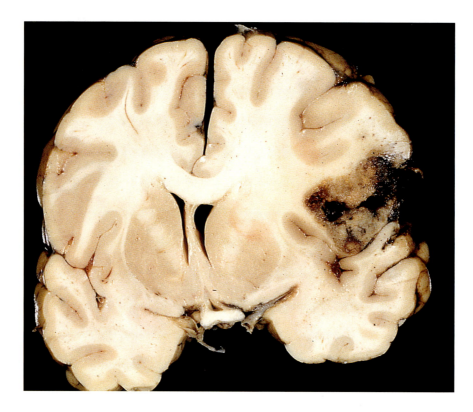

Figure 4.137 Cerebral secondaries. Coronal section of cerebrum at the level of the optic chiasm shows a well-defined intrinsic tumor with central necrosis. Cystic degeneration is present immediately above the right sylvian fissure. Carcinomas are characteristically well demarcated from the adjacent brain tissue

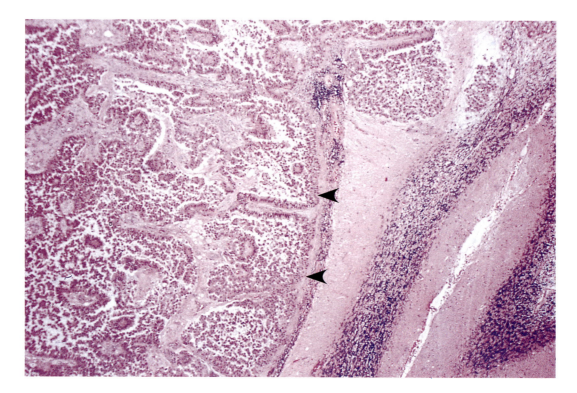

Figure 4.138 Cerebral secondaries. Histology of a metastatic adenocarcinoma in the cerebellum shows the disorganized papillary processes (arrowed) to be well differentiated from the surviving cerebellar cortical tissue. (H & E)

malformation, especially if they have bled or been treated surgically (Table 4.12).

Cerebral infarction

This probably accounts for one-third of all cases of epilepsy commencing after 60 years of age (Figures 4.143–4.145). A retrospective population-based study reported risks of early (less than 1 week) and late (more than 1 week) seizures to be 6.2% and 7.4%, respectively. Early seizures often occur within 24 h. Infarction in the anterior cerebral hemispheres and embolic events carry higher risks. Of the cases with late seizures, 73% occurred within 2 years of stroke.

Middle cerebral artery aneurysm

Unruptured aneurysms rarely cause seizures, but there is a high risk of epilepsy if they bleed and, in particular, after surgical treatment of a middle cerebral artery aneurysm (Figure 4.146).

Arteriovenous malformations

These are developmental anomalies which involve abnormal communications between the arterial and venous systems (Figure 4.147). The most common presentations are hemorrhage in approximately 50%,

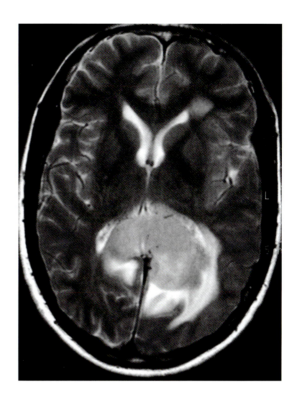

Figure 4.139 Primary CNS lymphoma. T2-weighted MRI axial image shows hyperdense mass straddling the midline posterior to the third ventricle in the region of the splenium of the corpus callosum. Note the perilesional white matter edema. This is typical of classical primary central nervous system lymphoma

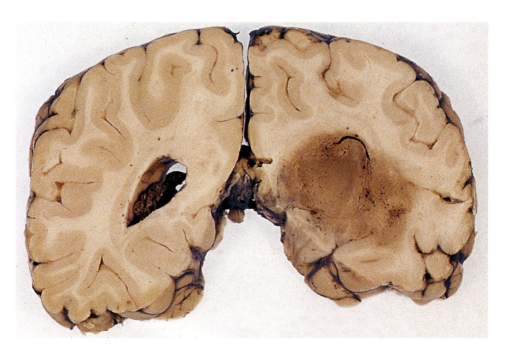

Figure 4.140 Primary cerebral lymphoma. Coronal section of cerebrum immediately posterior to the corpus callosum splenium shows an ill-defined diffusely infiltrating tumor adjacent to the right lateral ventricle. Primary cerebral lymphomas are often multiple, periventricular and ill-defined

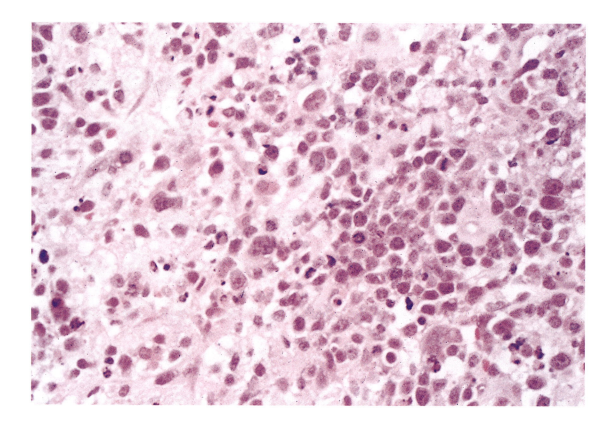

Figure 4.141 Primary cerebral lymphoma. Histology reveals that these are nearly always high-grade non-Hodgkin's B-cell lymphomas. They diffusely infiltrate the brain, but show accentuation of infiltration around blood vessels. (H & E)

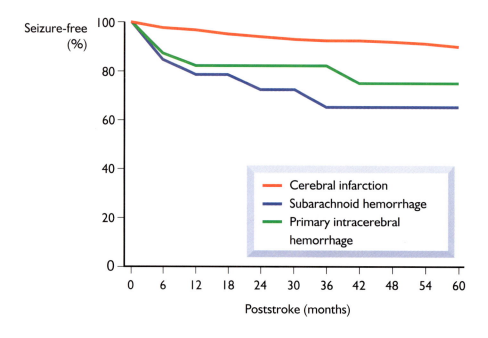

Figure 4.142 Risks of seizure after stroke. Modified from reference 8

Table 4.12 Non-malignant neurosurgical conditions and incidence of seizures. With permission from reference 9

Condition	Incidence of seizures (%)
Vascular	
anterior cerebral artery aneurysm	21
middle cerebral artery aneurysm	38
arteriovenous malformation	50
spontaneous hematoma	20
Meningioma	22
Abscess	92
Other benign supratentorial tumors	4
Shunting for hydrocephalus	17

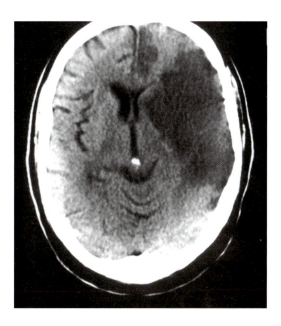

Figure 4.143 Middle cerebral artery infarct. A 72-year-old man had his first tonic-clonic seizure 1 year after he presented with a right hemiparesis. CT scan shows a right middle cerebral artery infarct

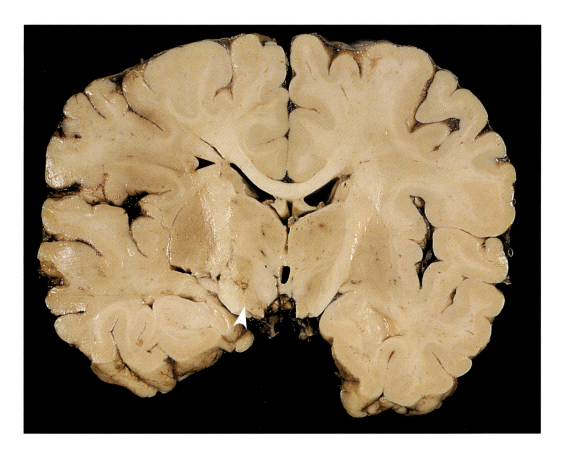

Figure 4.144 Recent cerebral infarct (ischemic). Coronal section of cerebrum shows the presence of a recent infarct in the left middle cerebral artery territory characterized by diffuse edema with blurring of the junction between gray and white matter. Ipsilateral tentorial herniation (arrowed) is evident

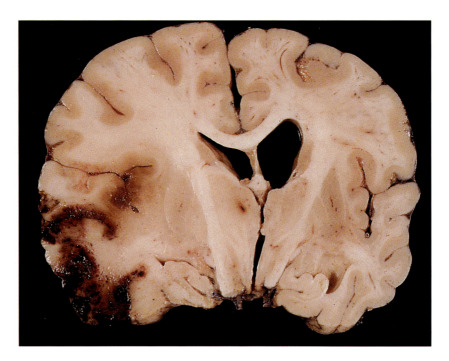

Figure 4.145 Recent cerebral infarct (hemorrhagic). Coronal section of cerebrum shows the presence of a recent hemorrhagic infarct in the overlap zone between the middle cerebral and posterior cerebral artery territories characterized by hemorrhage, most obvious in the gray matter. There is white matter edema, blurring of gray–white matter differentiation and conspicuous shift of midline structures from left to right, with ventricular compression and ipsilateral tentorial herniation. Hemorrhagic infarcts are due to the re-establishment of perfusion through devitalized brain tissue and may also be due to, for example, transient cerebral hypoperfusion or lysis of an embolus previously occluding a supplying artery

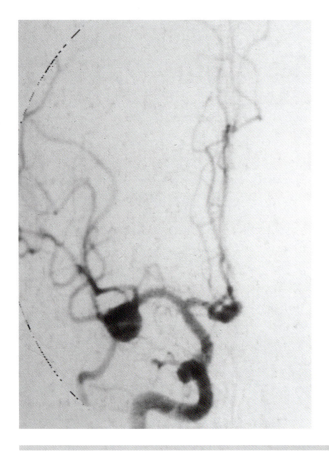

Figure 4.146 Middle cerebral artery aneurysm. Five days prior to hospital admission, a 68-year-old man developed a sudden severe headache and vomited. Physical examination and CT were normal, but cerebrospinal fluid was xanthochromic, and angiography revealed a large middle cerebral artery aneurysm and smaller right anterior communicating artery aneurysms. Because of his age, the presence of multiple lesions and the increased risk of epilepsy, the patient decided not to undergo surgery

seizures in 30%, chronic headache in 10% and progressive focal deficits in 7–10%. If untreated, the cumulative risk of hemorrhage is 1–4% per annum depending on the characteristics of the arteriovenous malformation (AVM). This risk increases to 6–18% in patients who present with a hemorrhage.

Of these lesions, 20–40% of AVMs are amenable to surgery, particularly those small superficial AVMs. Embolization can be effective therapy in up to 11%, or can be used to reduce the size of the nidus prior to definitive surgical treatment. Stereotactic radiosurgery is successful in selected patients, causing obliteration of 40% of AVMs at 1 year and 80% at 2 years. The main aim of any treatment of AVMs is to prevent future hemorrhage, but may also improve seizure control in a proportion of patients.

Venous sinus thrombosis

Occlusion of the cerebral venous sinuses is an uncommon cause of stroke. Most cases are idiopathic, but predisposing factors include local sepsis, disseminated malignancy, hypercoagulability states, the puerperium and, in babies and infants, dehydration.

The primary pathological event is cerebral infarction, but hemorrhage often supervenes. Clinical features vary according to the site of venous occlusion, with hemiplegia and seizures being a common presentation of sagittal sinus thrombosis. Diagnosis may be suspected on CT (Figure 4.148) and can be confirmed by angiography or non-invasively by MRI (Figure 4.149).

The overall mortality is 20–30% and is dependent on the underlying cause. A randomized controlled

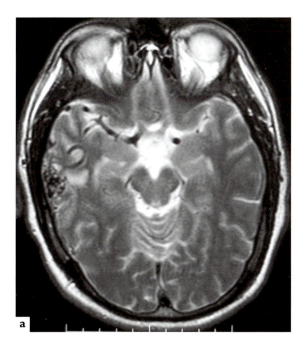

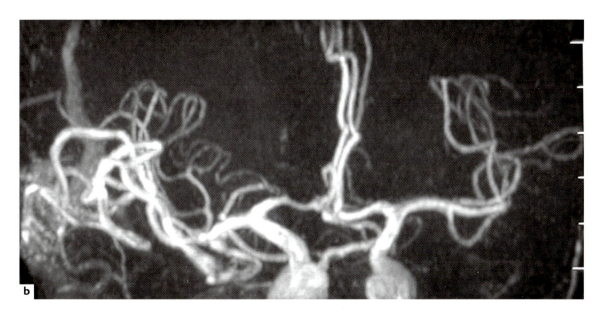

Figure 4.147 Arteriovenous malformation. A 42-year-old man began to experience simple partial seizures consisting of a stereotyped brief rising epigastric sensation. Following his first tonic-clonic seizure he had a contrast-enhanced CT and then MRI (a) and MR angiography (b) which confirmed a right temporal lobe arteriovenous malformation

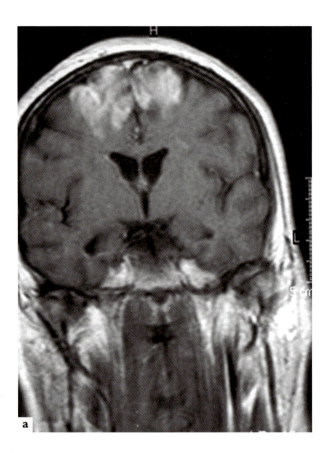

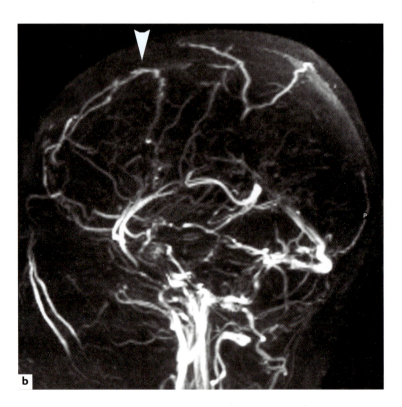

Figure 4.148 Sagittal sinus thrombosis. A 29-year-old woman who was 2 weeks' postpartum developed a subacute headache, and then had repeated tonic-clonic seizures several days later. She had bilateral papilledema. Coronal, T2-weighted MRI (a) shows bilateral parasagittal venous infarcts, and MR venogram (b) confirmed a sagittal sinus thrombosis (arrow)

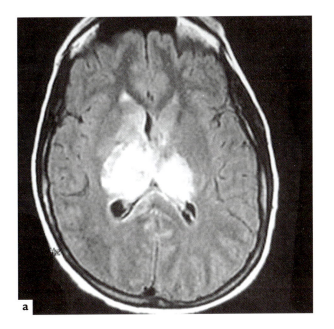

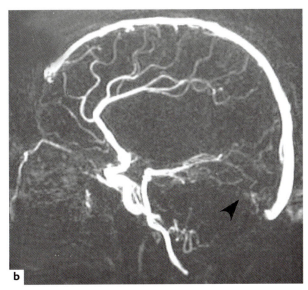

Figure 4.149 Straight sinus thrombosis. A 43-year-old woman presented in an acute confusional state. She was lethargic and disorientated, but had no focal neurological signs. MRI axial FLAIR (a) shows high signal throughout both thalami caused by inflammation secondary to venous infarction. The sagittal MR venogram (b) shows thrombosis of the straight sinus (arrow)

trial showed a non-statistically significant benefit of anticoagulation over placebo, even in patients with secondary cerebral hemorrhage[10]. The incidence of late epilepsy is not known.

Intracerebral hematoma

This is usually the consequence of moderate-to-severe hypertension. Hemorrhage is classified as massive, small or slight, with the prognosis directly related to size. Sites of predilection include the putamen, thalamus, pons, cerebellum and the occipital lobes. Patients with lobar hemorrhage (Figure 4.150) are more usually normotensive and an underlying arteriovenous malformation should be suspected. Seizures occur in 10–20% of cases.

Moya moya disease

This is a rare, non-inflammatory vasculopathy that may be uni- or bilateral resulting in an acute or, more commonly, chronic occlusion of the internal carotid arteries. The basilar artery is occasionally involved. Presentation is usually from 2 to 10 years of age with acute hemiparesis, or hemiplegia that may be transient or permanent; however, it can also occur in adolescence with transient ischemic attacks or subarachnoid hemorrhage. Seizures are a relatively

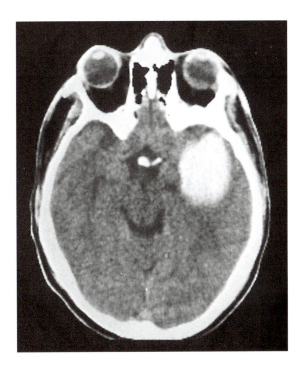

Figure 4.150 Intracerebral hematoma. A 17-year-old boy presented with an acute onset of headache, vomiting and aphasia. CT shows a hyperdense mass in the left temporal lobe, a small amount of surrounding low-density areas and a mass effect. At craniotomy, no arteriovenous malformation was identified, but a small lesion might have been obliterated by the bleed. Postoperatively, the patient has developed temporal lobe epilepsy

uncommon presentation and tend to occur in late childhood. Magnetic resonance angiography (MRA) or formal cerebral angiography demonstrate the extensive network of telangiectatic collateral vessels which develop over time following the carotid artery occlusion. The vessels resemble a blush or 'puff of smoke' from which the Japanese word 'moya moya' is derived (Figure 4.151).

Cerebral lupus

Systemic lupus erythematosus commonly involves the central nervous system. The cerebral manifestations are caused by widespread microinfarction due to arteriolar proliferation and destruction rather than by true vasculitis.

The clinical manifestations are protean, but seizures, cognitive and behavioral symptoms, and focal signs predominate. The CSF and CT scan are often normal, and MRI is the investigation of choice. Discrete and diffuse patterns of magnetic resonance abnormality can be identified, with the latter more commonly associated with seizures (Figure 4.152).

CADASIL

Cerebral autosomal dominant arteriopathy with subcortical infarcts and leucoencephalopathy (CADASIL) is an autosomal dominant condition characterized clinically by recurrent subcortical ischemic strokes, beginning usually in the fifth or sixth decade, and progressing to pseudobulbar palsy and dementia. Seizures can occur as part of the condition, but more common are psychiatric features

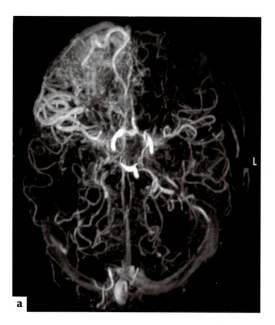

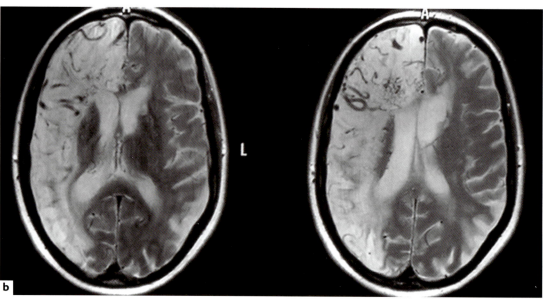

Figure 4.151 Moya moya disease. MR angiography (a) demonstrates occlusion of all major arteries distal to the circle of Willis with collateralization through a massive expansion of the basal capillary bed. Note the extreme hypervascularity of the right frontal region to the detriment of the right middle and posterior lobes which are rendered ischemic. The left frontal lobe is poorly served, but the middle and posterior lobes are more generously supplied. The T2-weighted image (b) shows high signal changes secondary to ischemia throughout most of the right hemisphere and some ischemic change in the deep left frontal lobe. Note signal voids of dilated vessels in right frontal region

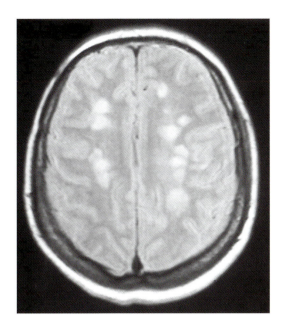

Figure 4.152 Cerebral lupus. A 49-year-old woman with a clear history of strokes affecting both vertebrobasilar and carotid territories presented with left focal motor seizures that responded to carbamazepine. Extensive vascular screening was normal with the exception of a strongly positive antidouble-stranded DNA antibody (1 : 1280). MRI reveals multiple periventricular high-intensity lesions

including mania or depression and migraine-like headaches.

MRI shows small deep infarcts and a leucoencephalopathy (Figure 4.153), and white matter hyperintensity in the temporal poles is specific for CADASIL compared with hypertensive changes. CADASIL is caused by a mutation in the notch 3 gene on chromosome 19q13.

Seizures and epilepsy following cardiac bypass surgery

Cardiopulmonary bypass surgery has increased in both sophistication and availability over the past decade. Total correction of previously inoperable congenital cardiac defects is being undertaken at progressively younger ages, and coronary artery and valve replacement is being performed in adults with increasing frequency.

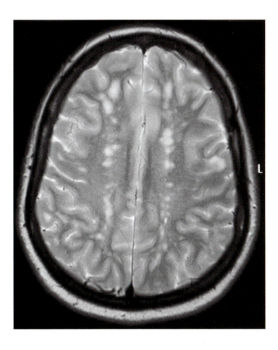

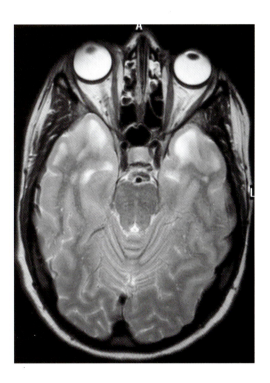

Figure 4.153 Cerebral autosomal dominant arteriopathy with subcortical infarcts and leucoencephalopathy (CADASIL). A 34-year-old woman presented with episodes of right-sided hemisensory disturbance and dysphasia, followed by severe throbbing headaches and photophobia with full recovery in between. Neurological examination was normal. Her maternal grandmother, and mother (and two of her siblings) had had strokes in their fifties or sixties. Her mother and two brothers had migraine, and one had had a transient ischemic attack at the age of 30. MRI scan shows multiple areas of high signal intensity in the subcortical white matter, and this also involves the anterior temporal lobe in a pattern typical for CADASIL. Genetic testing for CADASIL was positive for a mutation in the notch 3 gene

Although most patients undergo surgery without complications, neurological sequelae may occur as a consequence of microembolization, hypoxia, cerebral hypoperfusion (ischemia) and metabolic dysfunction (Figure 4.154). In addition to epileptic seizures, which are a common complication and may be either transient or persistent, non-epileptic movement disorders (usually chorea and athetosis) may also occur. Patients may develop both focal and generalized epileptic seizures. Focal seizures are often difficult to control and are refractory to antiepileptic drug treatment. Chronic epilepsy in these situations is frequently associated with neurological deficit (hemiplegia or quadriplegia) and cognitive dysfunction.

REFERENCES

1. Gutierrez-Delicado E, Serratosa JM. Genetics of the epilepsias. Curr Opin Neurol 2004; 17: 147–53

2. McKusick VA. Mendelian Inheritance in Man, 9th edn. Baltimore: Johns Hopkins University Press, 1990

3. Sisodiya SM. Malformations of cortical development: burdens and insights from important causes of human epilepsy. Lancet Neurol 2004; 3: 29–38

4. Janz D. Juvenile myoclonic epilepsy. In Dam M, Gram L, eds. Comprehensive Epileptology. New York: Raven Press, 1990: 171–85

5. Laidlaw J, Richens A, Chadwick D, eds. A Textbook of Epilepsy, 4th edn. London: Churchill Livingstone, 1993: 64

6. Chang BS, Lowenstein DH. Practice parameter: antiepileptic drug prophylaxis in severe traumatic brain injury. Report of the Quality Standards Subcommittee of the American Academy of Neurology. Neurology 2003; 60: 10–16

7. Sander JWAS, Hart YM, Johnson AL, Shorvon SD. National General Practice Study of Epilepsy: newly diagnosed epileptic seizures in a general population. Lancet 1990; 36: 267–71

8. Burn J, Sandercock P, Bamford J, et al. Epileptic seizures after first ever in a lifetime stroke. The Oxfordshire Community Stroke Project. Br Med J 1997; 315: 1582–7

9. Foy PM, Copeland GP, Shaw MDM. The incidence of post-operative seizures. Acta Neurochir 1981; 55: 253–64

10. de Bruijn SF, Stam J. Randomized, placebo-controlled trial of anticoagulant treatment with low-molecular-weight heparin for cerebral sinus thrombosis. Stroke 1999; 30: 484–8

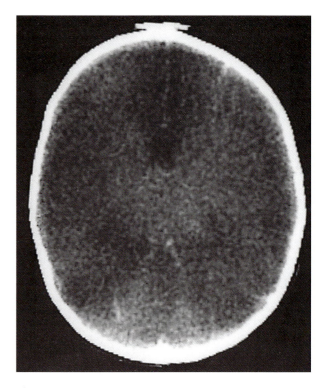

Figure 4.154 Postcardiac bypass surgery hypoxia. A 9-month-old child had a severe and prolonged hypotensive episode during cardiac bypass surgery and, upon recovery from the anesthetic, was found to be non-responsive and in status epilepticus. Axial CT shows cerebral edema with diffuse areas of low density bilaterally (more on the right than on the left) suggesting cerebral infarction. The patient survived with intractable epilepsy, spastic quadriplegia and cortical visual impairment

5. Prognosis

EPILEPSY

Prior to the availability of effective antiepileptic drugs, epilepsy was probably a chronic disabling condition in most cases. Even following the discovery of effective antiepileptic drugs, selected hospital-based statistics suggested a poor prognosis, with only approximately 30% of patients achieving remission (Table 5.1)[1].

In contrast, recent studies (Table 5.2)[2–16] in unselected populations have demonstrated a favorable outlook with up to 70% of patients achieving protracted remission (Figure 5.1).

Although the overall prognosis is good, 25–30% of patients continue to have seizures despite optimal drug therapy. This reflects the heterogeneity of the epilepsies and several biological variables that influence the prognosis in a given patient. Studies in unselected populations consistently identify a limited number of interdependent variables (Table 5.3) that characterize patients likely to develop a chronic condition. The prognosis of any patient with epilepsy is dependent on the underlying syndrome (Table 5.4) and/or its cause.

Table 5.1 Prognostic studies of chronic epilepsy. With permission from reference 1

Reference	n	Duration of remission (years)	Percentage in remission
Habermass (1901)	937	2	10
Turner (1907)	87	2	32
Grosz (1930)	125	10	11
Kirstein (1942)	174	3	22
Alstroem (1950)	897	5	22
Strobos (1959)	228	1	38
Kjorbe, Lund & Poulsen (1960)	130	4	32
Probst (1960)	83	2	31
Trolle (1960)	799	2	37
Juul-Jensen (1963)	969	2	32
Lorge (1964)	177	2	34

Table 5.2 Prognostic studies in newly diagnosed patients

Type of study	No. of patients	Type of study	Duration of remission (years)	Percentage in remission
Community (retrospective)				
Annegers et al., 1979[2]	457	A	5	70.0*
Goodridge and Shorvon, 1983[3]	122	C	4	69.0*
Hospital (retrospective)				
Okuma and Kumashiro, 1981[4]	1868	A	3	58.3
Shafer, 1988[5]	306	C	5	66.0
Camfield, 1996[6]	479	C	*	70.0
Hospital (prospective)				
Sofijanov 1982[7]	512	P	2	50.6
Elwes et al., 1984[8]	106	A	2	82.0*
Brorson, 1987[9]	194	P	3	64.0
Collaborative Group, 1992[10]	280	C	2	67.5*
Camfield, 1993[11]	504	P	2	70.0
Semah, 1998[12]	2200	A	1	45.0
Arts, 1999[13]	466	P	1	57.0
Berg, 2001[14]	613	P	1	53.0
Community (prospective)				
Cockerell, 1997[15]	792	C	3	86.0
Sillanpaa, 1998[16]	245	P	5	64.0

*Physician and family felt sufficient time seizure free to consider AED withdrawal determined by actuarial analysis
P, pediatric; A, adult; C, combination

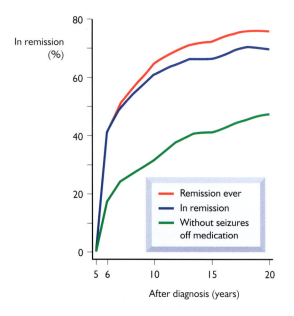

Figure 5.1 Percentage of patients achieving remission at 5 years or more during the first 20 years after diagnosis of epilepsy

Table 5.3 Adverse prognostic factors

Symptomatic etiology

Partial-onset seizures

Atonic seizures

Late-onset or first-year epilepsy

Additional mental or motor handicap

Long duration prior to treatment

Poor initial response to treatment

DRUG WITHDRAWAL

In a heterogeneous group of patients with epilepsy in remission, planned withdrawal of antiepileptic drugs doubled the risk of relapse at 2 years (Figure 5.2). Multivariate analysis demonstrated a limited number of independently significant prognostic variables

Table 5.4 Prognosis by epilepsy syndrome

Good

Benign neonatal familial convulsions

Childhood-onset absence epilepsy

Benign partial epilepsy with occipital paroxysms

    early onset (Panayiotopoulos syndrome)

    late onset (Gastaut syndrome)

Benign childhood epilepsy with rolandic spikes

Juvenile myoclonic epilepsy (but relapses common if

  treatment discontinued)

Epilepsy with grand mal on awakening

Intermediate

Benign myoclonic epilepsy of infancy

Juvenile-onset absence epilepsy

Myoclonic–astatic epilepsy

Poor

Ohtahara syndrome (early infantile epileptic encephalopathy)

West's syndrome

Severe myoclonic epilepsy in infancy (Dravet syndrome)

Lennox–Gastaut syndrome

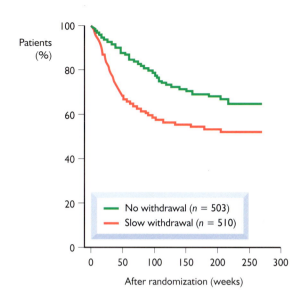

Figure 5.2 Actuarial percentage of patients remaining seizure-free with continued treatment compared with slow withdrawal of antiepileptic drugs. Modified with permission from reference 17

(Table 5.5). From these data, a predictive model has been developed from which a patient's risk of relapse at 1 and 2 years can be calculated.

SINGLE SEIZURES

Methodological differences explain the widely varying estimates of the risk of recurrence after an isolated seizure (Table 5.6). Meta-analysis of prospective studies, using first-seizure methods, indicates an overall 2-year risk of 30–40%.

Etiology and the EEG appear to be the most important predictors of recurrence. When these factors are combined, the lowest risk (24%) is in the idiopathic group with a normal EEG, and the highest risk (65%) is in remote symptomatic seizures associated with an epileptiform EEG.

The MESS study (MRC Multicentre study of Early epilepsy and Single Seizures) randomized 1443 patients who had experienced either a single unprovoked seizure or a small number of seizures to immediate or deferred treatment[17]. Patients randomized to deferred antiepileptic drug (AED) treatment received no drugs until such time as the clinician and patient agreed that treatment was unavoidable.

Table 5.5 Prognostic variables for recurrence after antiepileptic drug withdrawal. Adapted with permission from reference 17

Variable	RR	95% CI
Period seizure-free		
< 2.5 years	1.00	
2.5–< 3 years	0.94	0.67, 1.32*
3–< 5 years	0.67	0.48, 0.93*
5–< 10 years	0.47	0.32, 0.69*
History of partial seizures only	2.51	1.00, 6.30†
History of myoclonic seizures	1.85	1.09, 3.12†
History of tonic-clonic seizures	3.40	1.48, 7.84†
More than one antiepileptic drug at randomization	1.79	1.34, 2.39†
Seizures after start of treatment	1.57	1.10, 2.24†

*Factors associated with lower risk of relapse
†Factors associated with higher risk of relapse
RR, relative risk

Table 5.6 Prognosis for recurrence after 'first' seizures

Reference	n	Median follow-up	Time at which outcome was ascertained	Recurrence risk (%)
First-seizure methods				
Prospective ascertainment				
Austin et al., 2002[18]	224	2 years	2 years	73
Ramos Lizana et al. 2000[19]	133	—	5 years	64
Shinnar et al., 2000[20]	407	—	10 years	46
Stroink et al., 1998[21]	156	44 months	2 years	54
Martinovic et al., 1997[22]	78	>2 years	—	69
FIRST trial group, 1993[23]	193	> 2 years	2 years	51
Hauser et al., 1990[24]	208	> 2 years	5 years	34
Shinnar et al., 1991[25]	283	> 2.7 years	4 years	42
Camfield et al., 1989[26]	47	> 1 year	1 year	38
Hopkins et al., 1988[27]	306	—	4 years	52
Pearce & Mackintosh, 1979[28]	22	> 12 months	1 year	23
Retrospective ascertainment				
Hui et al., 2001[29]	132	—	3 years	47
Hart et al., 1990[30]	564	> 2 years	3 years	78
Boulloche et al., 1989[31]	119	> 5 years	8 years	38
Annegers et al., 1986[32]	424	> 2 years	5 years	56
Camfield et al., 1985[33]	168	2 years	2 years	52
Elwes et al., 1985[34]	133	15 months	3 years	71
Cleland et al., 1981[35]	70	4 years	—	39
Hyllested & Pakkenberg, 1963[36]	63	> 4 years	—	43
Thomas, 1959[37]	48	> 3 years	—	27
Saunders & Marshal, 1975[38]	39	2 years	—	33
New-onset epilepsy methods				
Prospective ascertainment				
Marson et al., 2005[39]	721	—	8 years	52
Ramos Lizana et al., 2000[19]	217	—	5 years	79
Blom et al., 1978[40]	74	3 years	3 years	58
Retrospective ascertainment				
Hertz et al., 1984[41]	435	to age 7	at age 7	69
van den Berg & Yerushally, 1969[42]	113	to age 5	at age 5	65

Immediate treatment reduced the risk of first seizure (hazard ratio (HR) 1.4 (95% CI 1.2 to 1.7)) and reduced the time to achieve a 2-year remission of seizures ($p = 0.023$). At 5 years, 76% of the immediate treatment and 77% of the deferred treatment group were in a 2-year terminal remission (difference –0.2% (95% CI –5.8%, 5.5%)) (Figure 5.3).

This is the largest published study to examine the question of the impact of early AED treatment. It provides evidence to suggest that although early

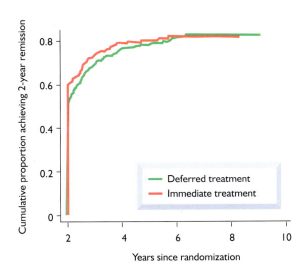

Figure 5.3 Cumulative proportion of patients achieving 2-year seizure remission following a single seizure. With permission from reference 39

treatment undoubtedly affects the short-term risk of recurrence, the long-term prognosis is unaffected. Unfortunately, there were limited pediatric data; additional and more comprehensive data have been made available from other population-based studies[19,20], including the excellent Dutch national study of epilepsy in childhood[21].

REFERENCES

1. Reynolds EH. The prognosis of epilepsy: is chronic epilepsy preventable? In Trimble MR, ed. Chronic Epilepsy, its Prognosis and Management. Chichester: John Wiley & Sons, 1989: 13–20

2. Annegers JF, Hauser WA, Elveback LR. Remission of seizures and relapse in patients with epilepsy. Epilepsia 1979; 20: 729–37

3. Goodridge DMG, Shorvon SD. Epileptic seizures in a population of 6,000. II. Treatment and prognosis. BMJ 1983; 287: 645–7

4. Okuma T, Kumashiro H. Natural history and prognosis of epilepsy: report of a multi-institutional study in Japan. Epilepsia 1981; 22: 25–53

5. Shafer SQ, Hauser WA, Annegers JF, Klass DW. EEG and other early predictors of epilepsy remission: a community study. Epilepsia 1988; 29: 90–600

6. Camfield CS, Camfield PR, Gordon K, Dooley J. Does the number of seizures before treatment influence ease of control or remission of childhood epilepsy? Not if the number is 10 or less. Neurology 1996; 464: 41–4

7. Sofijanov NG. Clinical evolution and prognosis in childhood epilepsies. Epilepsia 1982; 23: 61–9

8. Elwes RDC, Johnson AL, Shorvon SD, Reynolds EH. The prognosis for seizure control in newly diagnosed epilepsy. N Engl J Med 1984; 311: 944–7

9. Brorson LO, Wranne L. Long-term prognosis in childhood epilepsy: survival and seizure prognosis. Epilepsia 1987; 28: 324–30

10. Collaborative Group for the Study of Epilepsy. Prognosis of epilepsy in newly referred patients: a multicentre study of the effects of mono-therapy on the long-term course of epilepsy. Epilepsia 1992; 33: 45–51

11. Camfield CS, Camfield PR, Gordon K, Smith B, Dooley J. Outcome of childhood epilepsy: a population-based study with a simple scoring system for those treated with medication. J Pediatr 1993; 122: 861–8

12. Semah F, Picot M-C, Adam C, Broglin D, Arzimanoglou A, Bazin B, Cavalcanti D, Baulac M. Is the underlying cause of epilepsy a major prognostic factor for recurrence? Neurology 1998; 51: 1256–62

13. Arts WFM, Geerts AT, Brouwer OF, Peters ACB, Stroink H, van Donselaar CA. The early prognosis of epilepsy in childhood: the prediction of a poor outcome. The Dutch study of epilepsy in childhood. Epilepsia 1999; 40: 726–34

14. Berg AT, Shinnar S, Levy SR, Testa FM, Smith-Rapaport S, Beckerman B, Ebrahimi N. Two-year remission and subsequent relapse in children with newly diagnosed epilepsy. Epilepsia 2001; 42: 1553–62

15. Cockerell OC, Johnson AL, Sander JWAS, Shorvon SD. Prognosis of epilepsy: a review and further analysis of the first nine years of the British National General Practice Study of Epilepsy, a prospective population-based study. Epilepsia 1997; 38: 31–46

16. Sillanpaa M, Jalava M, Kaleva O, Shinnar S. Long-term prognosis of seizures with onset in childhood. N Engl J Med 1998; 338: 1715–22

17. MRC Antiepileptic Drug Withdrawal Study Group. A randomized study of antiepileptic drug withdrawal in patients in remission of epilepsy. Lancet 1991; 1: 1175–80

18. Austin JK, Dunn DW, Caffrey HM, et al. Recurrent seizures and behavior problems in children with first

recognized seizures: a prospective study. Epilepsia 2002; 43: 1564–73

19. Ramos Lizana J, Cassinello Garcia E, Carrasco Marina LL, et al. Seizure recurrence after a first unprovoked seizure in childhood: a prospective study. Epilepsia 2000; 41: 1005–13

20. Shinnar S, Berg AT, O'Dell C, et al. Predictors of multiple seizures in a cohort of children prospectively followed from the time of their first unprovoked seizure. Ann Neurol 2000; 48: 140–7

21. Stroink H, Brouwer OF, Arts WFM, et al. The first unprovoked, untreated seizure in childhood: a hospital based study of the accuracy of the diagnosis, rate of recurrence, and long term outcome after recurrence. Dutch study of epilepsy in childhood. J Neurol Neurosurg Psychiatry 1998; 64: 595–600

22. Martinovic Z, Jovic N. Seizure recurrence after a first generalized tonic-clonic seizure, in children, adolescents and young adults. Seizure 1997; 6: 461–5

23. First Seizure Trial Group (FIRST GROUP). Randomized clinical trial on the efficacy of antiepileptic drugs in reducing the risk of relapse after a first unprovoked tonic-clonic seizure. Neurology 1993; 43: 478–83

24. Hauser WA, Rich SS, Annegers JF, Anderson VE. Seizure recurrence after a first unprovoked seizure: an extended follow-up. Neurology 1990; 40: 1163–70

25. Shinnar S, Berg AT, Moshe SL, et al. The risk of recurrence following a first unprovoked seizure in childhood: a prospective study. Pediatrics 1991; 85: 1076–85

26. Camfield P, Camfield C, Dooley A, et al. A randomized study of carbamazepine versus no medication after a first unprovoked seizure in childhood. Neurology 1989; 39: 851–2

27. Hopkins A, Garman A, Clark C. The first seizure in adult life: value of clinical features, electroencephalography and computerised tomographic scanning in prediction of seizure recurrence. Lancet 1988; 1: 721–6

28. Pearce JL, Mackintosh HT. Prospective study of convulsions in childhood. NZ Med J 1979; 89: 1–3

29. Hart YM, Sander JWAS, Johnson AL, Shorvon SD. The National General Practice Study of Epilepsy: recurrence after a first seizure. Lancet 1990; 336: 1271–4

30. Hui AC, Tang A, Wong KS, et al. Recurrence after a first untreated seizure in the Hong Kong Chinese population. Epilepsia 2001; 42: 94–7

31. Boulloche I, Leloup P, Mallet E, et al. Risk of recurrence after a single unprovoked generalised tonic-clonic seizure. Dev Med Child Neurol 1989; 39: 626–32

32. Annegers JF, Shirts SB, Hauser WA, Kurland LT. The risk of recurrence after an initial unprovoked seizure. Epilepsia 1986; 27: 43–50

33. Camfield PR, Camfield CS, Dooley JM, et al. Epilepsy after a first unprovoked seizure in childhood. Neurology 1985; 35: 1657–60

34. Elwes RDC, Chesterman P, Reynolds EH. Prognosis after a first untreated tonic-clonic seizure. Lancet 1985; ii: 752–3

35. Cleland PG, Mosquera I, Stuard WP, Foster JB. Prognosis of isolated seizures in adult life. Lancet 1981; 2: 1364

36. Hyllested K, Pakkenberg H. Prognosis in epilepsy of late onset. Neurology 1963; 13: 641–4

37. Thomas MH. The single seizure – its study and management. JAMA 1959; 169: 457–9

38. Saunders M, Marshal C. Isolated seizures: An EEG and clinical assessment. Epilepsia 1975; 16: 731–3

39. Marson AG, Jacoby A, Johnson A, et al. for the Medical Research Council MESS study group. Immediate versus deferred antiepileptic drug treatment for early epilepsy and single seizures: a randomised controlled trial. Lancet 2005; 365: 2007–13

40. Blom S, Heijbel J, Bergfors PG. Incidence of epilepsy in children: a follow-up study three years after the first seizure. Epilepsia 1978; 19: 343–50

41. Hertz DG, Ellenberg JH, Nelson KP. The risk of recurrence of nonfebrile seizures in children. Neurology 1984; 34: 637–41

42. van den Berg BJ, Yerushally J. Studies on convulsive disorders in young children. Pediatr Res 1969; 3: 298–304

6. Management

MEDICAL TREATMENT

The first and most important aspect of treatment is to establish a correct diagnosis of epilepsy and the epilepsy syndrome or seizure type and to always consider a possible underlying cause; the second step is to decide that treatment with antiepileptic drugs is necessary; and the third is to decide which drug should be used. The choice of drug depends on the specific epilepsy syndrome or, if no syndrome has been identified, on the type of seizure or seizures experienced by the patient. Where there are two or three possible 'first-choice' drugs, the potential side-effects and formulation of the drug can be used to decide which might be the most suitable. In the future, the cause of the epilepsy or the identification of any specific drug-resistant genes in an individual patient may become the most important factor in helping to determine the choice of drug.

Figure 6.1 is a diagrammatic representation of the evolution of antiepileptic drugs over time. Most controlled studies have shown no clear benefit of one antiepileptic agent over another; the only obvious exception to this is the proven efficacy of sodium valproate in juvenile myoclonic epilepsy.

Table 6.1 outlines the antiepileptic drugs commonly prescribed in the most frequent types of adult and childhood epilepsy. Table 6.2 lists some of the antiepileptic agents currently under investigation. Patients and their families should receive counseling regarding:

(1) Aims of treatment;

(2) Prognosis and duration of the expected treatment;

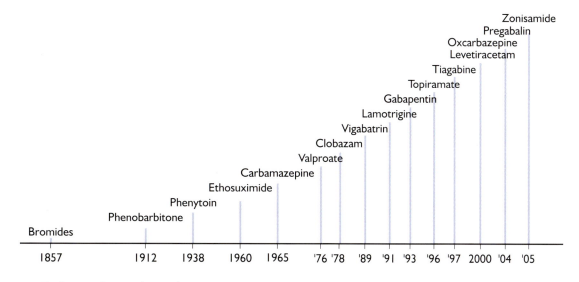

Figure 6.1 Evolution of antiepileptic drug treatment over time

Table 6.1 Most commonly prescribed antiepileptic drugs for the most common types of adult and childhood epilepsy (listed in alphabetical order and not in order of preference)

Epilepsy syndrome or seizure type	Commonly used drug
Idiopathic (primary) generalized, including typical absence, juvenile myoclonic, tonic-clonic seizures on awakening	clobazam/clonazepam*
	ethosuximide (absences)
	lamotrigine
	levetiracetam[†]
	sodium valproate
	topiramate[††]
Myoclonic–astatic, myoclonic seizures (benign or progressive) and atonic seizures	clobazam/clonazepam
	ethosuximide
	lamotrigine
	sodium valproate
	stiripentol[‡]
	topiramate
	zonisamide
Localization-related (idiopathic/symptomatic), including benign 'rolandic', benign 'occipital' and secondarily generalized seizures	acetazolamide
	carbamazepine
	gabapentin
	lamotrigine
	levetiracetam
	oxcarbazepine
	phenytoin
	sodium valproate
	tiagabine
	topiramate
	vigabatrin
	zonisamide
Lennox–Gastaut syndrome	clobazam
	lamotrigine
	sodium valproate
	topiramate
Infantile spasms (West's syndrome)[†††]	immunoglobulin (i.v.)
	nitrazepam
	prednisolone/ACTH (tetracosactide)
	sodium valproate
	vigabatrin

*The benzodiazepines (clonazepam and nitrazepam more than clobazam) are frequently restricted by tachyphylaxis and tolerance
[†]Early data suggest that levetiracetam may be effective in treating primary generalized tonic-clonic and myoclonic seizures
[††]Topiramate demonstrates little efficacy in treating typical absence seizures
[‡]Stiripentol is effective in treating the myoclonic (and, possible, the other seizure types) in severe myoclonic epilepsy of infancy
[†††]There remains a difference of opinion in the first-choice treatment of infantile spasms between Europe and the USA. In Europe the usual drug of first-choice is vigabatrin (despite the concern over the bilateral visual field constriction associated with this drug), whilst in USA the preferred drug is ACTH or prednisolone[l]

Table 6.2 New antiepileptic drugs

Drug	Mode of action
Eterobarbital	?increased GABA inhibition
Loreclezole	not known
Losiganone	?enhancement of GABA-mediated inhibition
Ralitoline	?inactivation of voltage-dependent sodium channel
Remacemide	non-competitive NMDA antagonist

(3) Importance of compliance adherence;

(4) Side-effects.

Ideally, patients/parents should be given written information on both any epilepsy syndrome identified in the individual and the drug prescribed which should provide the following information:

(1) Available preparations of the drug;

(2) Dosing schedule;

(3) Method of administration (particularly important for children);

(4) What to do if a dose is missed or vomited;

(5) Which other drugs (including over-the-counter medicines) can be safely given with the antiepileptic drug(s);

(6) Likely and potential adverse side-effects and what to do if they are experienced.

The initial dose of the chosen drug should be the lowest possible that will achieve seizure control. If necessary, the dose should be increased gradually to the maximum clinically tolerated level (irrespective of serum levels) before abandoning its use and transferring the patient to another drug.

Approximately 70% of all patients with epilepsy enter prolonged remission with monotherapy. Comparative studies indicate little difference in efficacy among the commonly used conventional drugs. However, carbamazepine is probably the drug of choice for partial-onset seizures and, despite the absence of controlled data (except in juvenile myoclonic epilepsy), valproate is accepted as the drug of choice for generalized-onset seizures.

There is little evidence of success with dual therapy after failure of optimal doses of a single antiepileptic drug; indeed, seizure control may improve after switching from dual therapy to monotherapy. Furthermore, any improvement in seizure control attributable to the addition of a second drug may be at the expense of increased toxicity.

Complete seizure control with or without evidence of major toxicity is never achieved by at least 25% of patients. Such patients frequently require a therapeutic compromise (determination of a personalized balance between seizure control and adverse effects). In this group of patients, new antiepileptic drugs or surgery, or both, should be considered.

Meta-analyses of published randomized controlled trials of novel antiepileptic drugs as add-on therapy suggest that lamotrigine and gabapentin are 2.5–3.0 times, and tiagabine and vigabatrin 5–6 times, and levetiracetam and topiramate 7–8 times more likely than placebo to produce a 50% or greater reduction of seizures. The apparently greater efficacy of topiramate appears to be at the expense of greater toxicity. However, whether or not these findings are genuine or spurious requires direct comparisons between these compounds. Such a comparative study has recently been completed in the UK – the SANAD study (Standard And New Antiepileptic Drugs). This randomized study comprised of two arms: one comparing the 'standard' drug, sodium valproate against the newer drugs lamotrigine and topiramate; the other comparing the 'standard' drug, carbamazepine against the newer drugs, gabapentin, lamotrigine, oxcarbazepine and topiramate in approximately 2500 patients aged 5 years and above in both partial (focal) and generalized seizures and epilepsy syndromes. The results of this largest yet conducted randomized study of antiepileptic drugs in children and adult patients with epilepsy are extremely interesting and will be published in mid to late 2006 in *The Lancet*.

Monitoring the serum levels of antiepileptic drugs is often undertaken, but is only of limited practical use. The therapeutic or target ranges are only guidelines as the optimal level for any given patient may lie well above or below these ranges. In most cases, the dosage of antiepileptic drug is considered appropriate when the patient is seizure-free with no (or at least patient-acceptable) side-effects. Antiepileptic drug levels should be measured in patients who present with status epilepticus, in patients suspected of major non-adherence, or in those receiving polytherapy which includes phenytoin.

Table 6.3 Acute anticonvulsant toxicity with antiepileptic drug treatment

Dose-related	
Encephalopathy (tiredness, nystagmus, ataxia, dysarthria, confusional state)	phenytoin, carbamazepine, phenobarbitone, benzodiazepines, lamotrigine, gabapentin, sodium valproate
Movement disorder	phenytoin
Tremor	valproate
Idiosyncratic	
Hypersensitivity	phenytoin, carbamazepine, phenobarbitone, lamotrigine
Aplastic anemia	carbamazepine, phenytoin, felbamate
Acute hepatitis	valproate, phenytoin, phenobarbitone, felbamate
Acute psychosis	vigabatrin, topiramate
Complex partial status epilepticus	tiagabine

Side-effects of antiepileptic drug treatment

Adverse effects with antiepileptic drugs are common. The risk of acute dose-related symptoms and acute idiosyncratic reactions (Table 6.3) can be minimized by cautious dose escalation. Chronic toxicity (Table 6.4) and teratogenicity (Table 6.5) are directly related to high-dose polytherapy.

Some reactions, however, cannot be easily assigned to any of these categories. Incidental mechanisms of action can be important; for example, paresthesia and renal calculi are probably due to the carbonic anhydrase activity of topiramate and zonisamide. Acute psychotic reactions have a multifactorial basis and rarely represent idiosyncratic toxicity.

A non-specific dose-related encephalopathy is common, predictable and reversible. Valproate-induced tremor is common at high doses, whereas phenytoin on rare occasions produces a dose-dependent dyskinesia.

Acute idiosyncratic reactions are rare, unpredictable and require immediate drug withdrawal. The risk of hypersensitivity reactions, manifested by rash with or without fever (Figures 6.2–6.4), ranges from 2 to 4%, whereas Stevens–Johnson syndrome occurs in 1 : 5000–10 000 patients exposed to carbamazepine, phenytoin, phenobarbitone or lamotrigine. Aplastic anemia is an extremely rare

Table 6.4 Chronic anticonvulsant toxicity with antiepileptic drug treatment

Nervous system
Memory and cognitive impairment, hyperactivity and behavior disturbances, pseudodementia, cerebellar atrophy, peripheral neuropathy, appetite stimulant (particularly with sodium valproate) and appetite suppressant (particularly topiramate)

Eyes
Bilateral visual field constriction (vigabatrin); glaucoma (topiramate)

Skin
Acne, hirsutism, alopecia, chloasma

Liver
Enzyme induction

Blood
Megaloblastic anemia, thrombocytopenia, pseudolymphoma

Immune system
IgA deficiency, drug-induced systemic lupus erythematosus

Endocrine system
Decreased thyroxine levels, increased cortisol and sex hormone metabolism

Bone
Osteomalacia

Connective tissue
Gingival hypertrophy, coarsened facial features, Dupuytren's contracture

Table 6.5 Teratogenicity of antiepileptic drug treatment

Fetal anticonvulsant syndrome	phenytoin, valproate, trimethadione
Spina bifida	valproate (1–2%), carbamazepine (0.5–1%)

complication of phenytoin or carbamazepine therapy, whereas acute liver failure attributable to valproate is seen almost exclusively in children < 2 years of age with additional, and usually severe, development delay. Felbamate carries significant risk of fatal hematological or hepatic reactions.

Chronic exposure to antiepileptic drugs can affect any system. A reversible peripheral neuropathy, cerebellar atrophy and osteomalacia are unusual problems essentially confined to institutionalized patients. Cosmetic side-effects attributable to phenytoin or phenobarbitone are particularly troublesome in young women. Gingival hypertrophy is seen in one-third of patients receiving phenytoin (Figure 6.5), developing after between 3 and 4 months of chronic exposure. Vigabatrin has been shown to be associated with bilateral viral field constriction in approximately one in three adults treated with this drug for at least 2 years; the incidence in

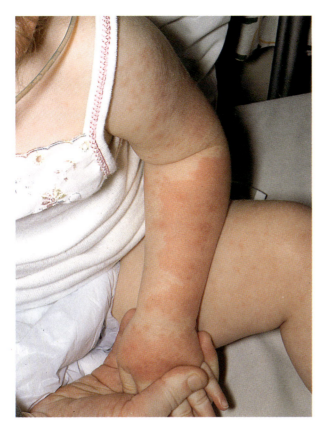

Figure 6.2 Lamotrigine rash. Six days after lamotrigine was added to her sodium valproate treatment, this 3-year-old girl with myoclonic epilepsy developed a widespread maculopapular rash accompanied by fever, malaise, vomiting and peripheral eosinophilia. The rash resolved within 1 week and recurred when she was 'challenged' with very low-dose lamotrigine 6 months later

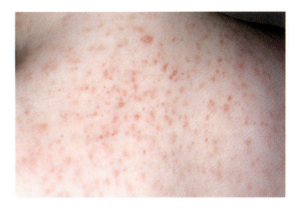

Figure 6.3 Lamotrigine rash. Five days after lamotrigine was added to his sodium valproate treatment, this 7-year-old boy with Lennox–Gastaut syndrome developed a widespread papular rash associated with low-grade fever which resolved within 10 days

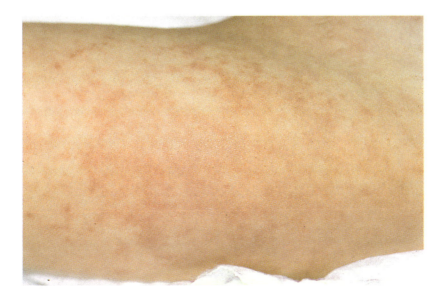

Figure 6.4 Phenytoin rash. Following a near-drowning accident, an 8-year-old boy was in a coma. A diffuse fine maculopapular rash appeared 48 h after he received a loading dose of phenytoin for seizures. The patient was receiving no other medication

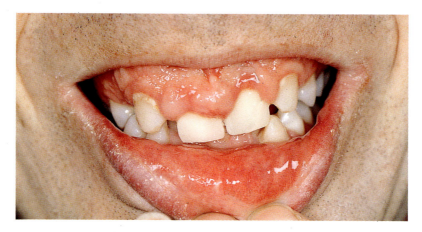

Figure 6.5 Phenytoin gingival hypertrophy. Moderate gingival hypertrophy has developed in this 32-year-old patient with chronic (2-year) phenytoin therapy

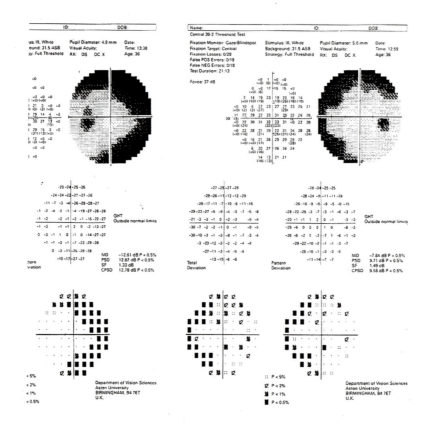

Figure 6.6 Vigabatrin-related visual field defect. A 28-year-old man with drug refractory temporal lobe epilepsy had been treated with a combination of carbamazepine and vigabatrin for the previous 4 years. He did not complain of any visual symptoms, but visual field testing revealed an asymptomatic binasal loss typical of a vigabatrin-related visual field defect. Vigabatrin was withdrawn, and subsequent testing was unchanged with the visual field defect remaining asymptomatic

children is not known but is considered to be lower, possibly affecting one in four children (Figure 6.6). There are conflicting data about the permanency of this visual field deficit; the deficit may be reversible in children.

Women with epilepsy account for 0.5% of all pregnancies. The overall risk of congenital malformations is 4–6%, but is significantly greater in mothers receiving high-dose polytherapy (Figures 6.7 and 6.8). A variety of congenital malformations have been reported in children born to mothers taking antiepileptic drugs (Table 6.6).

A non-specific fetal anticonvulsant syndrome manifested by orofacial clefts, distal digital anomalies (Figure 6.9) and mild mental handicap with or without cardiac defects has been attributed to several compounds. The risks of neural tube defects with valproate and carbamazepine are 1–2% and 0.5%, respectively. More recent data have suggested that children born to mothers taking sodium valproate (as mono- or polytherapy) appear to be at risk from developmental delay and, specifically, speech and language difficulties even in the absence of any major or minor congenital anomalies.

Although novel drugs are not recommended for pregnant patients, their thorough preclinical evaluation and early clinical data suggest less teratogenicity than with conventional drugs. It must be emphasized, however, that uncontrolled epilepsy presents greater risks than drug therapy to both pregnancy and fetal development.

Holistic management

The management of epilepsy extends far beyond the prescription of antiepileptic medication. For many patients and their families, the social, educational and psychological factors clearly outweigh the issue of seizure control. These needs should be met through a multidisciplinary approach that is preferably carried out within a specialist clinic (for

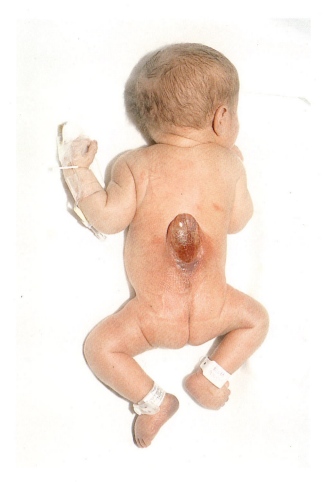

Figure 6.7 Spina bifida. A mother who had received sodium valproate and carbamazepine during pregnancy gave birth to an infant who had a low thoracic meningocele with no clinical or radiological evidence of hydrocephalus

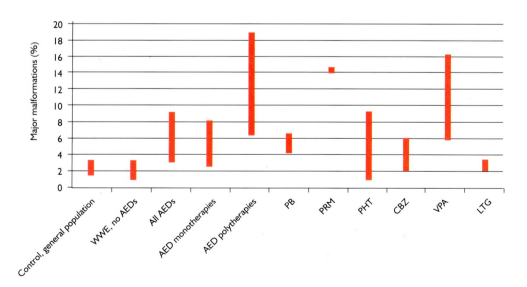

Figure 6.8 Overall mean major malformation (%) rates in children born to women with epilepsy (WWE), and the rates with the most commonly studied antiepileptic drug (AED) monotherapies. PB, phenobarbital; PRM, primidone; PHT, phenytoin; CBZ, carbamazepine; VPA, valproate; LTG, lamotrigine. With permission from reference 2

121

Table 6.6 Most commonly reported major malformations reported by specific AED exposure. With permission from reference 2

Type of AED	Neural tube defects (NTDs)	Oral clefts	Cardiac malformations	Urogenital defects (hypospadias)
PB		+	+	
PHT		+	+	±
PRM		+	+	
CBZ	+ 1%; OR of NTDs, 6.9 (CI 1.9–25.7)		+	+
LTG	+	+	+	+
VPA	+ 3.8%		+	+

OR, odds ratio; CI, 95% confidence interval; PB, phenobarbital; PHT, phenytoin; PRM, primidone; CBZ, carbamazepine; LTG, lamotrigine; VPA, valproate

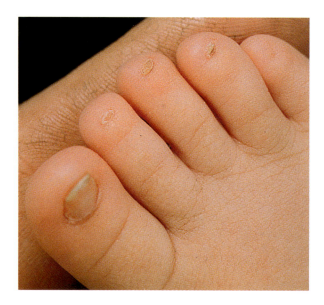

Figure 6.9 Fetal hydantoin syndrome. A 12-month-old infant, born to a mother with epilepsy who received phenytoin during pregnancy, has hypoplasia of the toenails (as well as of the fingernails), a well-recognized feature of this syndrome

Table 6.7 Multidisciplinary approach to the management of epilepsy

Dedicated trained and specialist medical staff

Clinical nurse specialist in epilepsy

Clinical psychologist

Psychiatrist

Social worker

Representatives of relevant voluntary associations and career advisers

Secretarial staff

both pediatric and adult patients) with access to education, support and advice from a number of different sources (Table 6.7) Recently published guidelines make this point and emphasize the non-drug management of all people with epilepsy[3,4].

Status epilepticus

Status epilepticus (SE) can be defined as recurrent epileptic seizures lasting more than 30 min. Although this definition of '30 min duration' has not yet been formally revised, there is a consensus that this should be re-defined to 5 min, based on data suggesting that spontaneous cessation of a tonic-clonic seizure was unlikely after 5 min (adults) and 10 min (children). In view of this it is generally agreed and recommended that any person who has been convulsing for more than 5 min should be regarded as being in convulsive status epilepticus and treated appropriately. A practical classification includes the following seizure types:

(1) Tonic-clonic;

(2) Absence (typical and atypical (Figure 6.10));

(3) Myoclonic;

(4) Complex partial (Figure 6.11);

(5) Focal motor (epilepsia partialis continua);

(6) Hypsarrhythmia (as in West's syndrome).

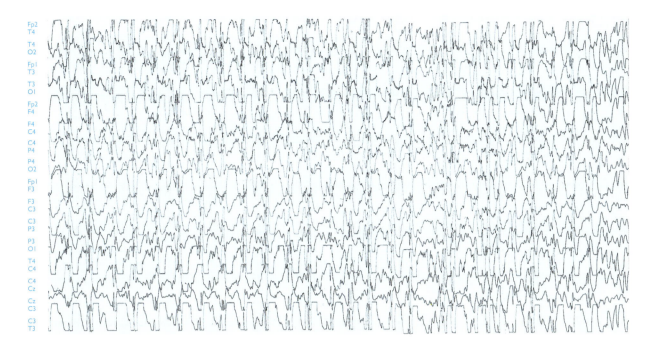

Figure 6.10 Atypical absence status epilepticus. A 10-year-old boy with Lennox–Gastaut syndrome presented with a 24-h history of confusion, unresponsiveness and semipurposeful movements. Awake EEG shows continuous irregular spike and slow-wave activity

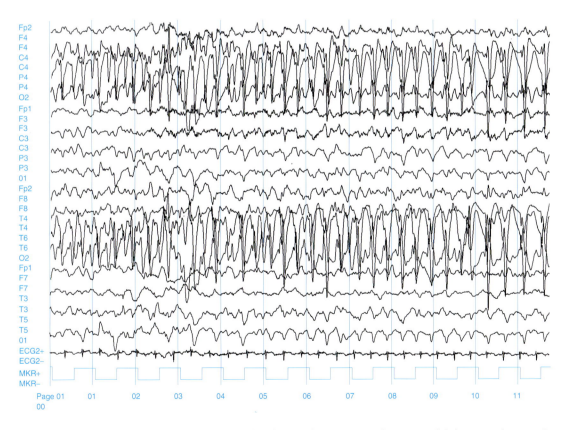

Figure 6.11 A 9-year-old girl who, following two brief partial seizures with temporal lobe semiology and, prior to commencing antiepileptic medication, presented in complex partial status epilepticus. Her EEG showed continuous right-sided (temporal/centrotemporal) rhythmic spike and slow-wave activity. The patient responded to a single dose of intravenous lorazepam and has remained seizure-free on low-dose carbamazepine. Cerebral MRI was normal. *Continued*

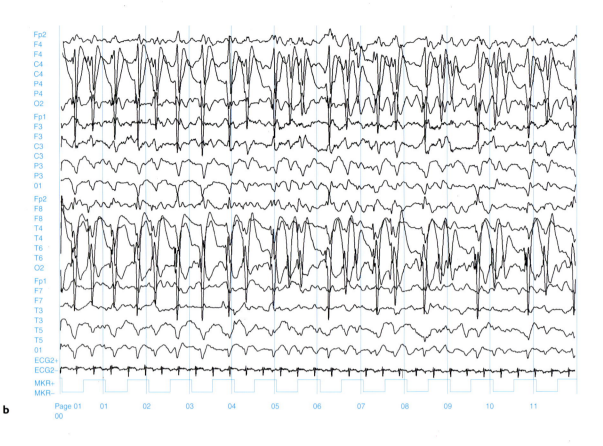

b

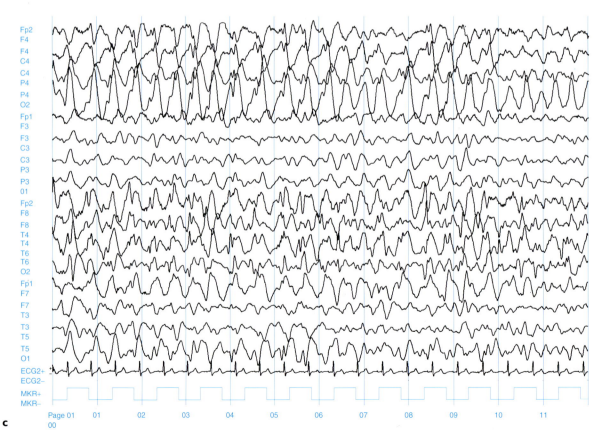

c

Figure 6.11 *Continued*

Tonic-clonic (also called convulsive) status epilepticus (CSE) is a common medical emergency which can be caused by any cerebral pathology, but the causes differ between children and adults (Table 6.8). CSE produces a characteristic pattern of changes which, ultimately, cause irreversible brain damage and potentially fatal systemic complications.

Table 6.8 Causes of tonic-clonic status epilepticus in children and adults

Children	Adults
Idiopathic (unknown)	non-adherence with anticonvulsants
Febrile	
Acute illness	alcohol
meningitis	drug overdose
encephalitis	stroke
head trauma	
	metabolic
Chronic epilepsy: acute exacerbation, acute anticonvulsant withdrawal or non-adherence with anticonvulsants	tumor
	infection
	unknown
Progressive encephalopathy	

During the first 30 min, compensatory mechanisms ensure that the delivery of glucose to active cerebral tissue is maintained but, when decompensation ensues, worsening systemic hypotension fails to satisfy the demands of cerebral tissue.

The aims of management are cessation of seizures, prevention of complications and treatment/reversal of the underlying cause (Figures 6.12 and 6.13). The process of management should be in phases which reflect the underlying pathophysiology (Table 6.9).

In early SE (< 30 min), intravenous benzodiazepine abolishes seizures in 70% of cases with a 10–15% rate of hypotension/respiratory depression. In most cases lorazepam has largely become the drug of first choice because of its rapid onset of action. Midazolam administered into either the buccal cavity or nostrils has become a useful and effective drug, and route of administration[6]. In the UK, buccal midazolam is now replacing rectal diazepam as the preferred non-intravenous method of giving a benzodiazepine, both in and out of hospital; this route is also preferred by carers and nursing staff in special schools and long-stay residential institutions. Rectal paraldehyde is occasionally used when patients are either resistant or sensitive to benzodiazepines.

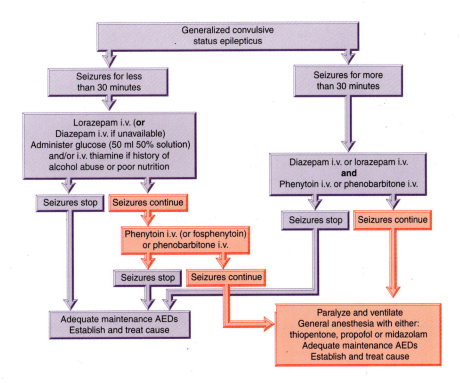

Figure 6.12 Recommended drug treatment for status epilepticus for adults

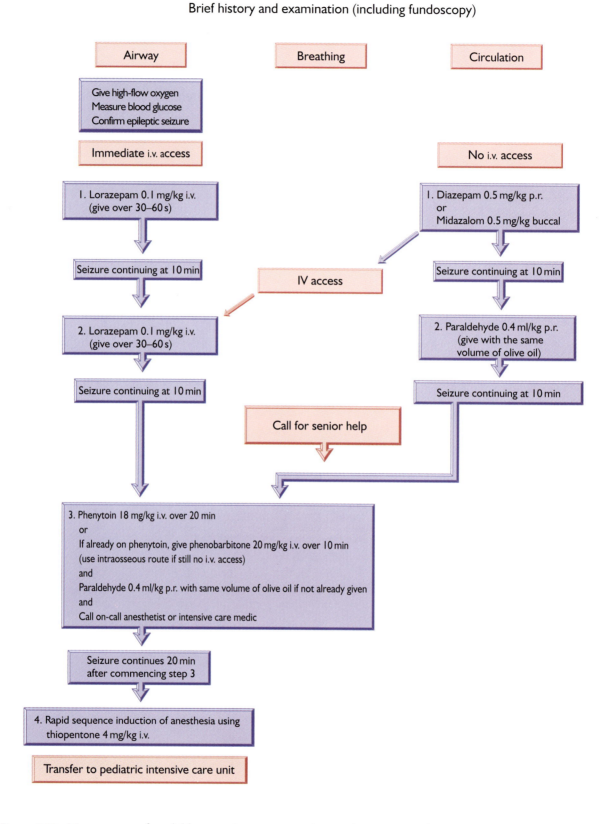

Brief history and examination (including fundoscopy)

Airway

Breathing

Circulation

Give high-flow oxygen
Measure blood glucose
Confirm epileptic seizure

Immediate i.v. access

No i.v. access

1. Lorazepam 0.1 mg/kg i.v.
(give over 30–60 s)

1. Diazepam 0.5 mg/kg p.r.
or
Midazalom 0.5 mg/kg buccal

Seizure continuing at 10 min

IV access

Seizure continuing at 10 min

2. Lorazepam 0.1 mg/kg i.v.
(give over 30–60 s)

2. Paraldehyde 0.4 ml/kg p.r.
(give with the same
volume of olive oil)

Seizure continuing at 10 min

Seizure continuing at 10 min

Call for senior help

3. Phenytoin 18 mg/kg i.v. over 20 min
or
If already on phenytoin, give phenobarbitone 20 mg/kg i.v. over 10 min
(use intraosseous route if still no i.v. access)
and
Paraldehyde 0.4 ml/kg p.r. with same volume of olive oil if not already given
and
Call on-call anesthetist or intensive care medic

Seizure continues 20 min
after commencing step 3

4. Rapid sequence induction of anesthesia using
thiopentone 4 mg/kg i.v.

Transfer to pediatric intensive care unit

Figure 6.13 Management of a child presenting to an accident and emergency department in an acute tonic-clonic convulsion including established convulsive status. Modified from reference 5

Table 6.9 Management of tonic-clonic status epilepticus (SE)

Stage of SE	Treatment	
	First choice	Alternatives
Early (0–30 min)	lorazepam i.v./p.r. midazolam buccal* diazepam i.v./p.r.	rectal paraldehyde
Established (30–60 min)	phenytoin i.v.† fosphenytoin i.v. phenobarbitone i.v.	
Refractory (60–90 min)	thiopentone i.v. pentobarbitone i.v.	propofol i.v. midazolam i.v.

*Buccal midazolam is replacing rectal diazepam in the UK
†Fosphenytoin i.v. has replaced phenytoin in the USA
p.r., per rectum, an important alternative route of administration in children when intravenous access is difficult or impossible

In established SE (30–60 min), the patient should be transferred to an intensive care unit (ICU) or an emergency treatment unit (ETU). The benzodiazepine midazolam can also be given as an infusion. Phenobarbitone possesses several advantages, but the prodrug fosphenytoin avoids the tissue-irritant and cardiotoxic effects of phenytoin, whilst retaining the rapid onset of action of phenobarbitone.

Patients in refractory SE (60–90 min) require ventilation with full ICU or ETU support. The intravenous barbiturates thiopentone and pentobarbitone are the drugs of first choice in these cases. However, although effective, both are associated with unfavorable pharmacokinetics and significant toxicity. The non-barbiturate anesthetic propofol is increasingly being used in adults on ICU/ETU; however, its use in children is much more limited owing to concerns over the development of the potentially fatal propofol infusion syndrome. The relative merits of these different approaches have not yet been determined. Nonetheless, whichever of these means is adopted, the continuation of usual antiepileptic drug therapy is essential.

SURGICAL TREATMENT

Surgical intervention is now accepted as a realistic therapeutic option for many patients with medically refractory seizures. Recent advances in presurgical investigation protocols and operative techniques

Table 6.10 Surgical procedures for refractory seizures

Functional surgery
Stereotactic lesions
  subcortical
  temporal
Disconnection procedures
  corpus callosotomy
    multiple subpial transections

Resective surgery
Temporal lobe resections
  neocorticectomy
  anterior temporal lobectomy
  amygdalohippocampectomy
Extratemporal resections
  frontal
  centroparietal
  occipital
Major resections
  multilobar
  hemispherectomy

Other
Vagal nerve stimulation
Deep brain stimulation (thalamus, basal ganglia)

have resulted in a rapid expansion in the number of neuroscience centers performing epilepsy surgery in both Europe and the USA. As a consequence, the number of successfully treated patients continues to rise steadily, although fewer surgical procedures are being undertaken globally based on the number of patients (of all ages) with drug-resistant epilepsy who could benefit from this therapeutic option.

Of the most commonly performed procedures (Table 6.10), the resective procedures are intended to be curative, whereas functional operations are essentially palliative. The results of temporal lobe resection are more favorable than extratemporal resection but, in either case, the outcome is dependent on underlying pathology.

Functional procedures

Corpus callosotomy (Figure 6.14) is the most 'commonly' performed palliative procedure. By disconnecting the epileptogenic cortex from the rest of the brain, damaging secondarily generalized seizures, which are associated with falls, may be abolished in up to 80% of cases, although, frequently, the results

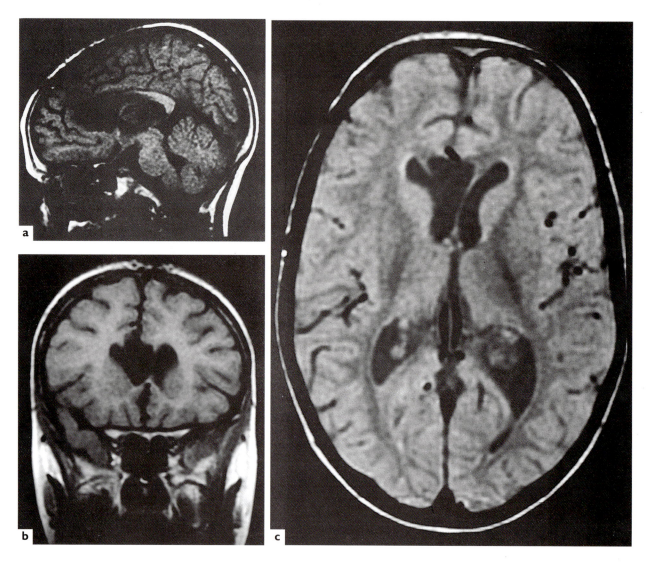

Figure 6.14 Corpus callosotomy. A 6-year-old boy who had Lennox–Gastaut syndrome experienced daily atonic and tonic seizures that were resistant to antiepileptic drug therapy. Parasagittal (a), coronal (b) and axial (c) MRIs were taken 2 months after sectioning of the anterior two-thirds of the corpus callosum. The atonic and tonic seizures resolved, but the partial seizures increased in frequency

are far less successful than this. A complex neuro-psychological deficit, the disconnection syndrome, can be prevented by anterior resection with sparing of the splenium. The incidence of other sequelae varies, but usually represents exacerbation of pre-existing deficits.

Resective procedures

Hemispherectomy

This dramatic procedure (Figure 6.15) is reserved for patients who have a congenital hemiplegia with no useful hand function and refractory seizures,

Sturge–Weber syndrome in which the hemiparesis is typically progressive, usually in association with frequent and drug-resistant seizures and, particularly (but not exclusively), in children with Rasmussen's 'encephalitis' (more appropriately termed Rasmussen's syndrome). Complete and sustained remission may be expected in 70–80% of patients. Improvement in contralateral motor function, intellect and behavior may also occur (Figures 6.16 and 6.17). A serious delayed complication, cerebral hemosiderosis, occurred in 25–33% of patients after anatomical hemispherectomy, but this problem has been overcome by modified (functional) procedures.

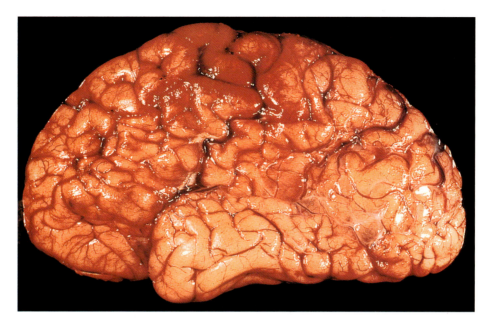

Figure 6.15 Hemispherectomy. External view of the left cerebral hemisphere shows areas of old ischemic damage particularly in the middle cerebral–posterior cerebral arterial boundary zone

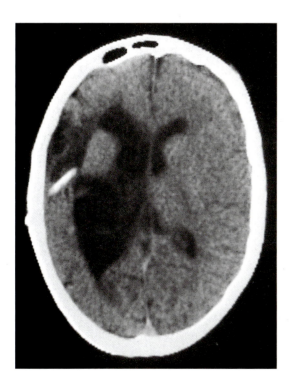

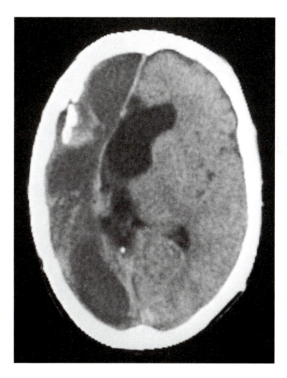

Figure 6.16 Hemispherectomy. A small boy had a congenital right hemiparesis, and refractory complex partial and secondarily generalized tonic-clonic seizures from the age of 1 year. Preoperative CT shows a shunt in a left temporal arachnoid cyst, left hemisphere atrophy and compensatory hydrocephalus. Postoperatively, he had an intracerebral hemorrhage, disseminated intravascular coagulation and oliguric renal failure

Figure 6.17 Hemispherectomy. Subsequent CT (same patient as in Figure 6.16) demonstrates the left hemispherectomy with a low-density collection in the left hemicranium and areas of calcification within this zone, probably representing organization of thrombus. Fortunately, the patient recovered fully and has been seizure-free for at least 2 years; he is able to walk unaided, his verbal communication skills have improved and he has learned to write

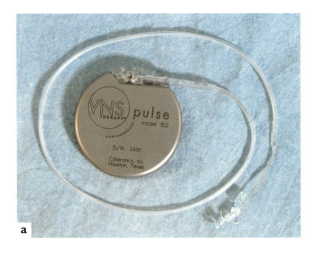

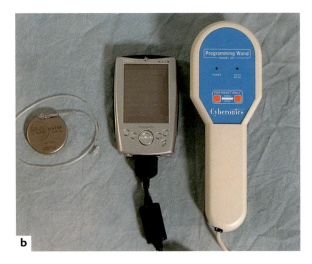

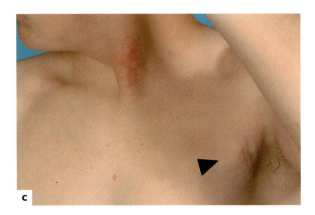

Figure 6.18 (a) The currently used vagal nerve stimulator (VNS Therapy™ Pulse Model 102, Cyberonics; Houston, Texas, USA) as used in our institution. (b) The stimulator with Programming Wand and the palmtop with software package. (c) A close-up of a patient with vagal nerve stimulator *in situ*. The implanted stimulator lies beneath the skin close to the left axilla (arrow)

Focal resections

The temporal lobe is the most common source of refractory partial seizures. A relatively homogeneous electroclinical temporal lobe 'syndrome' with a specific pathological substrate (Ammon's horn sclerosis) has been identified. This is not the case for extratemporal seizures. Unlike seizures of frontal lobe origin, temporal lobe seizures are easy to lateralize and, unlike the parietal and occipital lobes, the temporal lobe can be removed with relative impunity. Consequently, temporal lobe resections account for approximately two-thirds of all operations performed for intractable epilepsy and are associated with a better postoperative outcome than are extratemporal resections (75–80% vs. 50–60% seizure-free outcomes, respectively).

Vagal nerve stimulation

An increasingly used treatment for drug-resistant epilepsy, when there is no other surgical option (resection or disconnection), is vagal nerve stimulation (VNS)[7,8]. The mechanism by which stimulation of the vagus nerve leads to seizure inhibition is uncertain. Activation of afferent pathways from the nucleus solitarius of the vagus nerve to the thalami may produce an antiepileptic effect by suppressing rhythmic EEG activity. A programmable generator resembling a cardiac pacemaker is implanted beneath the left clavicle with electrodes wrapped round the left vagus nerve (Figure 6.18). The lifespan of the battery is generally 6–7 years, depending on the amplitude and rate of stimulation and how often an externally applied magnet is used to temporarily increase the rate of stimulation. Over 13 000 patients have been treated since the first one was implanted in 1989. Limited randomized controlled trial data suggest that approximately 40% of patients demonstrate a greater than 50% reduction in seizure frequency. Unfortunately, the antiseizure effect of VNS may not be obvious until at least 6–12 months following its implantation. As yet, it remains to be determined which seizure types (and epilepsy syndromes) will show the best response and how early a VNS should (and could) be implanted in children.

Deep brain stimulation

Although established as a treatment for patients with refractory Parkinson's disease, dystonia and tremor, it is still a new and largely experimental technique for patients with refractory epilepsy[9]. Areas stimulated have included the cerebellum, thalami (predominantly the anterior thalamic nuclei), caudate nuclei and temporal lobe. Data are very limited and, as yet, there is no information on the longer-term outcome of patients treated with this technique.

Temporal lobe surgery

There are no accurate estimates of the number of patients who might benefit from temporal lobe surgery. However, the available epidemiological data (Table 6.11) suggest that, in the UK, there is a reservoir of approximately 16 000 patients who have a history consistent with Ammon's horn sclerosis and that approximately 1000 new patients per year may present with this condition. In addition, there are likely to be several thousands of patients with definable structural abnormalities, mainly slow-growing and developmental tumors and focal cortical dysplasias.

Presurgical evaluation

Suitability for temporal lobe resection requires lateralization of seizure onset by imaging and EEG techniques, and exclusion of predictable surgical risks by neuropsychological examination. Although conventional CT scanning can detect gross pathology, this modality has been rapidly and wholly superseded by MRI, which is superior in detecting small structural and atrophic lesions. Asymmetry of medial temporal structures, demonstrated by MRI-based hippocampal volumetry, is highly correlated with histopathology and postoperative outcome. Postoperative MRI (Figure 6.19) is a useful method of demonstrating the completeness of resection.

Positron emission tomography (PET) scanning demonstrates hypometabolism in epileptic foci interictally and is a reliable indicator of the site of epileptogenic lesions. However, PET scanners are expensive to install and operate, and ictal events are not easily recorded with this technique. Consequently, this modality is not likely to become generally available. HMPAO–SPECT (hexamethylpropylene amine oxide–single-photon emission computed tomography) scans reveal hypoperfusion in epileptic foci interictally and hyperperfusion postictally. Comparison of interictal and ictal SPECT images (Figure 6.20) is highly predictive of the seizure focus. In some centers, concordance between interictal EEG, MRI, SPECT and psychometry obviates the need for invasive ictal monitoring

Table 6.11 Surgical procedures for refractory seizures

	$n/10^5$ population annually	Case total (n)
Prevalence		
Active epilepsy		400 000
Complex partial seizures		160 000
Drug-resistant CPS		80 000
with history of prolonged early 'febrile' convulsions		16 000
Incidence		
All new cases of epilepsy	50	30 000
Complex partial seizures	20	12 000
Likely to prove refractory	10	6000
with history of prolonged early 'febrile' convulsions	2	1200

CPS, complex partial seizures

Computer-aided subtraction ictal SPECT co-registered to MRI (SISCOM) is a technique that can reliably locate the epileptogenic zone by subtracting normalized and co-registered ictal and interictal SPECT images and then matching the resultant difference to high resolution MRI for anatomical correlation (Figure 6.21).

This technique may also be of value in deciding on the placement of depth (intracerebral) electrodes when investigating seizures of extratemporal origin.

Functional MRI (fMRI) is becoming established as a very useful imaging modality in many presurgical assessment programs and may replace SPECT and PET in presurgical evaluation programs (Figures 6.22–6.24). fMRI is an accurate method of lateralizing language function and therefore can complement the intracarotid amobarbital test in the process of presurgical evaluation. In the future fMRI may also become established in the assessment of memory functioning in this setting.

EEG remains the primary means of preoperative localization. A well-localized interictal anterior temporal spike focus (Figure 6.25) provides useful localizing information. However, bilateral independent spike foci are common and unilateral foci may be falsely lateralizing. Multicontact foramen ovale electrodes (Figure 6.26) are a useful means for lateralizing seizures with suspected medial temporal onset (Figure 6.27). However, if invasive EEG recordings are required to localize seizure-onset, then depth

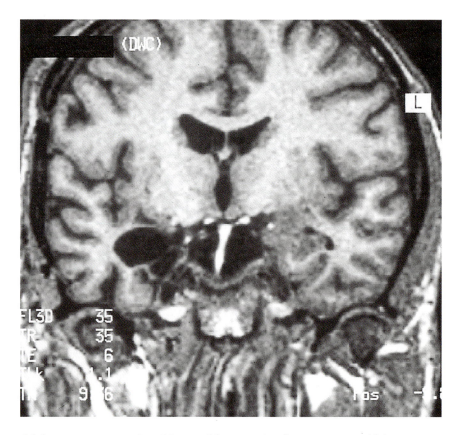

Figure 6.19 Amygdalohippocampectomy. In a 38-year-old man with refractory temporal lobe seizures, presurgical investigations demonstrated absent right-hemisphere memory function and a right medial temporal seizure onset. Postoperative MRI shows a low-signal area isointense with cerebrospinal fluid, on the medial surface of the right temporal lobe; such changes are typically seen after this operation

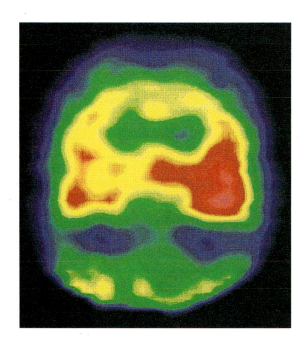

Figure 6.20 Seizures of medial temporal origin. Ictal HMPAO-SPECT scan shows left temporal hyperperfusion extending into the basal ganglia and adjacent frontal lobe, a typical pattern seen in these seizures

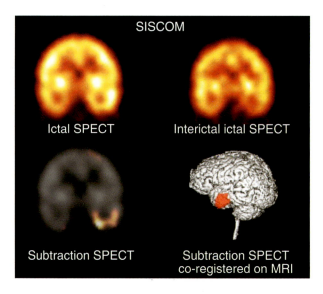

Figure 6.21 Ictal SPECT co-registered to MRI (SISCOM). SISCOM in a patient with right temporal lobe epilepsy. Routine MRI was normal. Note that the right side of the brain is on the right side of the figure

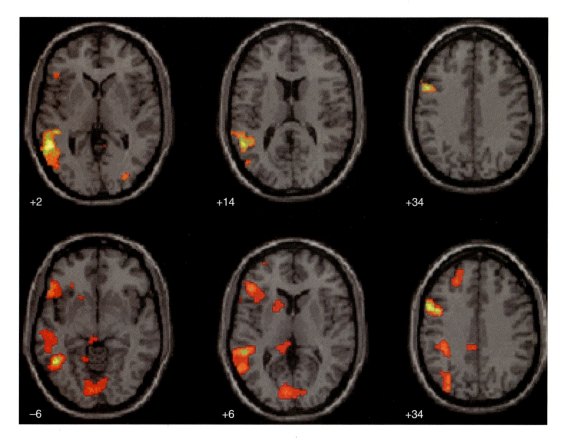

Figure 6.22 Functional magnetic resonance imaging. A 37-year-old man with right frontal lobe epilepsy focus; the tasks of listening to stories (upper images) and naming to description (lower images), shows left frontal and left temporal activation demonstrating left hemisphere dominance for language. Note that the left side of the image is the left brain

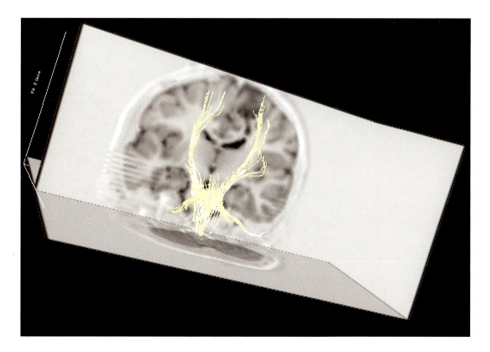

Figure 6.23 White matter tracts mapped around a left superior frontal gyrus tumor. The course of bilateral corticospinal tracts is demonstrated in relation to the tumor. Three-dimensional tractography was obtained following a 16 direction diffusion tensor acquisition on a 3 Tesla MR scanner

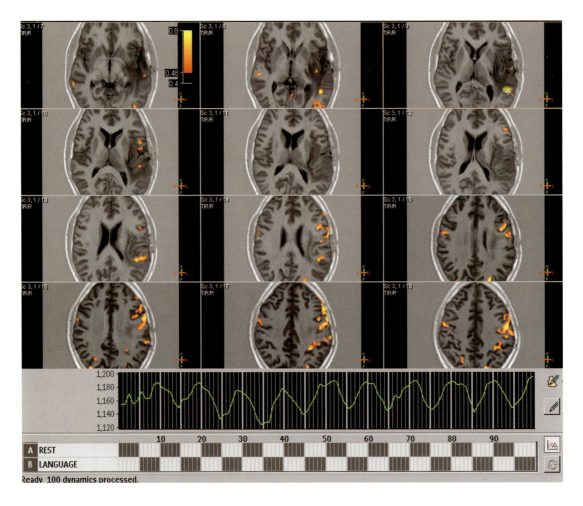

Figure 6.24 Functional MRI study using a word generation language paradigm. Left hemisphere language dominance is demonstrated. Language areas were mapped in relation to the tumor prior to planned resection of the left temporal lobe tumor. Study was carried out on a 3Tesla MR scanner

(Figure 6.28) and subdural electrodes (as grids or mats) are more accurate and allow the recording of activity from large areas of cortex. Cortical stimulation and electrocorticography may also provide valuable information when trying to define the extent (and limits) of any resection, particularly in extratemporal resections involving eloquent (functionally important) areas of cortex.

SURGICAL PATHOLOGY

Hemispherectomy

The distribution of pathologies for which hemispherectomy is performed is changing with time. Whereas early series were dominated by atrophic lesions secondary to infection or vascular accidents,

hemimegalencephaly, Sturge–Weber syndrome and Rasmussen's syndrome are currently the most common underlying lesions justifying hemispherectomy.

Focal resections

There is a broad spectrum of pathological substrates underlying focal epilepsy (Table 6.12). Formerly, extratemporal lesions were almost exclusively post-traumatic or postinfective scars (Figure 6.29) or tumors with a relatively high proportion of aggressive lesions, whereas temporal lobe resections usually revealed Ammon's horn sclerosis or indolent tumors. More recently, reports reveal an increasing proportion of developmental anomalies, the most common of which is focal cortical dysplasia (Figures 4.102, 4.103 and 6.30), most frequently found in frontal and central regions. Vascular malformations (Figures

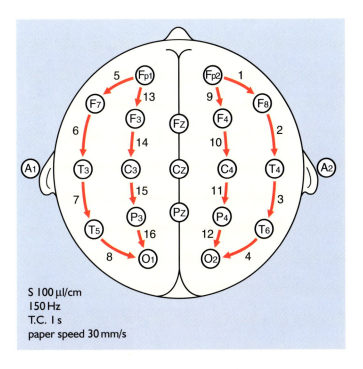

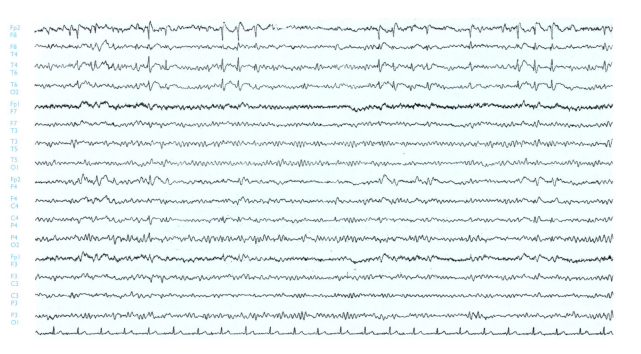

Figure 6.25 EEG shows a well-localized interictal right anterior temporal spike focus

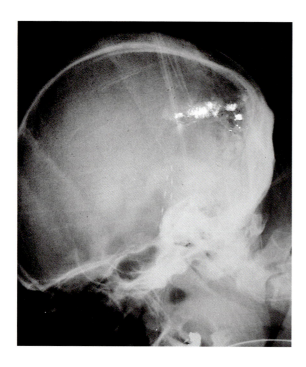

Figure 6.26 Lateral skull X-ray showing the position of multicontact foramen ovale electrodes. This is a useful means of lateralizing medial temporal seizures, but may provide misleading information if seizures originate elsewhere

6.31–6.33), which can arise at any site, account for a small proportion of cases of temporal lobe epilepsy.

The terminology used to describe the neuropathology of temporal lobe epilepsy has, until recently, been very confusing. However, improved surgical techniques allowing preservation of hippocampal specimens and advances in histopathological diagnosis have contributed to the production of an acceptable classification system (Table 6.13).

Ammon's horn sclerosis

Classical Ammon's horn sclerosis involves varying degrees of neuronal cell loss and gliosis in the CA1 and CA4 regions of the hippocampus and dentate gyrus (Figures 6.34 and 6.35). The condition is the cause of approximately 20% of cases of all refractory temporal lobe epilepsy. Ammon's horn sclerosis also accounts for 22–70% of cases in large surgical series. The variability may be due to presurgical selection, but the disorder is consistently the most common entity.

There is strong epidemiological and histopathological evidence to link prolonged early 'febrile' convulsions and Ammon's horn sclerosis. Although some authors contend that the relationship is definitely causal, it is equally likely that the severity of the 'febrile' convulsions and the refractory complex partial seizures are symptomatic of prenatally acquired cerebral damage, or even subtle dysplasia. It is also likely that a number of 'febrile' seizures are not temperature-related but are, in fact, unprovoked epileptic seizures.

The CT scan is often normal, but hippocampal atrophy and mesial temporal sclerosis can be readily detected by MRI (Figures 6.36 and 6.37). The degree of hippocampal asymmetry can be calculated using volumetric studies. Postoperatively, two-thirds of patients are rendered seizure-free and it has been suggested that diffuse sclerosis, involving the posterior hippocampus, is associated with a poorer outcome.

Neoplastic conditions

Indolent or very slow-growing tumors are reported in 13–56% of large surgical series. Their increased representation in recent reports probably reflects the wider availability of high-quality MRI. Although these lesions have similar radiological appearances, this category is pathologically heterogeneous, with relatively benign lesions predominating because of their propensity to cause refractory partial seizures. Low-grade gliomas (astrocytoma, oligodendroglioma), mixed cell tumors and anaplastic gliomas account for 60–70%, 20–30% and 10% of cases, respectively.

The mixed cell tumors have a limited growth potential and may not be truly neoplastic. The most common lesion, ganglioglioma (Figures 6.38 and 6.39), rarely undergoes malignant transformation. Dysembryoplastic neuroepithelial tumors (DNET) have become increasingly recognized, as a cause of refractory complex partial seizures with onset before age 20 years in neurologically normal individuals who have no evidence of a neurocutaneous syndrome. Their intracortical location is best determined by MRI (Figure 6.40).

The pathology of these tumors consists of glial nodules, foci of cortical dysplasia and a unique glioneuronal component with a characteristic appearance (Figures 6.41 and 6.42). They may resemble both ganglioglioma and true astrocytoma, but distinction from the latter can be made on both clinical and radiological grounds. At least 80% of patients are rendered seizure-free after resection of these lesions.

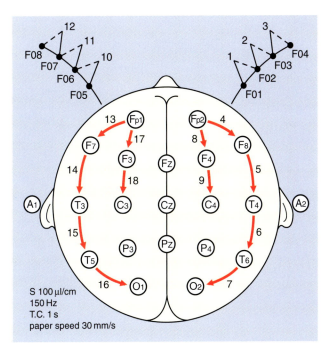

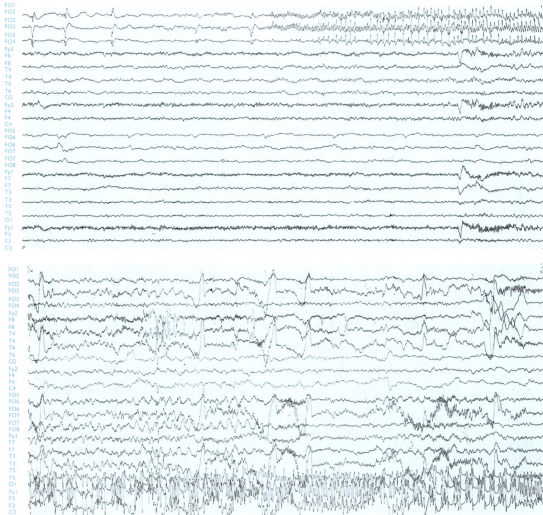

Figure 6.27 EEGs show lateralization of seizures of right medial temporal onset

Table 6.12 Structural lesions associated with epilepsy

Malformative

Cortical dysplasia

  microdysgenesis (Meencke)

  focal dysplasia

  cortical dysplasia with hamartomatous proliferation of
      neuroectodermal cells

  polymicrogyria

  lissencephaly/pachygyria

  hemimegalencephaly

Vascular malformations

  arteriovenous

  cavernous hemangioma

Neoplastic

Glioma

Ganglioglioma

Meningioma

Metastatic tumor

Dysembryoplastic neuroepithelial tumor (DNET)

Other

Familial and metabolic

With focal lesions; phakomatosis

  tuberous sclerosis

  neurofibromatosis

  encephalotrigeminal angiomatosis, Sturge–Weber syndrome

With diffuse lesions

  lysosomal enzyme deficiencies

  peroxisomal disorders

  mitochondrial enzyme disorders

  unknown etiology, e.g. Alexander's disease, lipofuscinosis,
      myelinopathies

Lafora body disease

Miscellaneous (often progressive) myoclonic epilepsies

Cerebrovascular disease and trauma

Ischemic

Hemorrhagic

Post-traumatic

Inflammatory/infectious

Fulminant encephalitis, e.g. due to herpesvirus

Chronic, e.g. parasitic

Rasmussen's 'encephalitis' (syndrome)

Ammon's horn (hippocampal) sclerosis

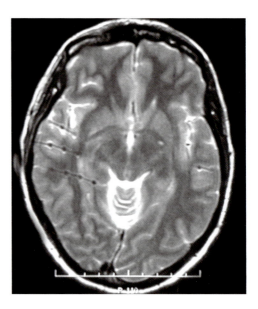

Figure 6.28 Depth electrodes. A 25-year-old man had complex partial seizures preceded by a stereotyped olfactory aura. MRI was normal, and ictal scalp EEG recordings had suggested the seizures had a right temporal onset. This was confirmed with depth electrode recordings, with three electrodes placed in the right temporal lobe and one in the left temporal lobe

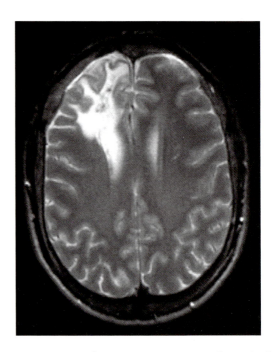

Figure 6.29 Postinfective scar. At 12 years of age, this boy underwent surgical drainage of a right frontal abscess. He then developed partial and tonic-clonic seizures 2 years later. MRI reveals high-signal, predominantly in the white matter of the anterior part of the right hemisphere, associated with enlargement of the right frontal horn. The central low-signal area suggests calcification. This is due to extensive gliosis around an old abscess cavity

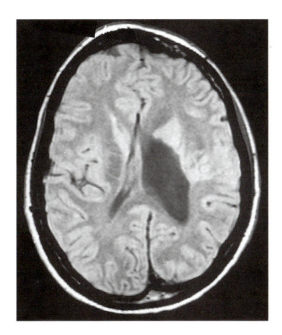

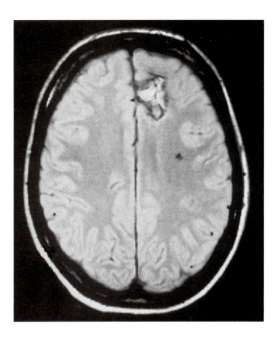

Figure 6.30 Cortical dysplasia. A 26-year-old woman had drug-resistant complex partial seizures with a right somatosensory aura, and right hemi-facial atrophy. MRI shows marked asymmetry of the hemispheres, with enlargement of the left lateral ventricle and a mass of heterotopic gray matter adjacent to the wall of the dilated ventricle. This is the typical appearance of dysplastic brain tissue in association with a neuronal migration disorder

Figure 6.31 Cavernous angioma. A highly intelligent child developed partial seizures manifested by speech arrest, confusion and bilateral motor automatisms with occasional secondary generalization. Axial MRI with T2 coronal and proton density demonstrates a partly serpiginous lesion in the left medial frontal region

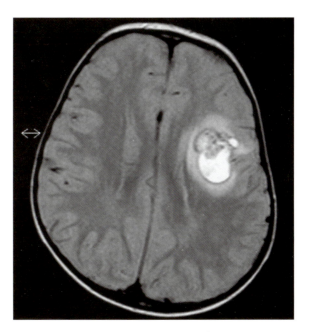

Figure 6.32 Cavernoma. A 23-month old boy (identical twin) presented at 21 months of age with frequent complex partial seizures affecting his head and right arm lasting approximately 1 minute and followed by speech arrest lasting 10 minutes. EEG demonstrated a persistent left central/centroparietal slow-wave discharge. Axial, T1-weighted MRI demonstrates a large lesion consistent with a hematoma surrounded by a rim of lower signal intensity (edema). There was no enhancement following intravenous gadolinium. Cerebral angiography and repeat MRI confirmed the presence of a cavernous hemangioma. The child has been seizure free for 15 months on no antiepileptic medication and with no motor or apparent cognitive deficit following surgical resection

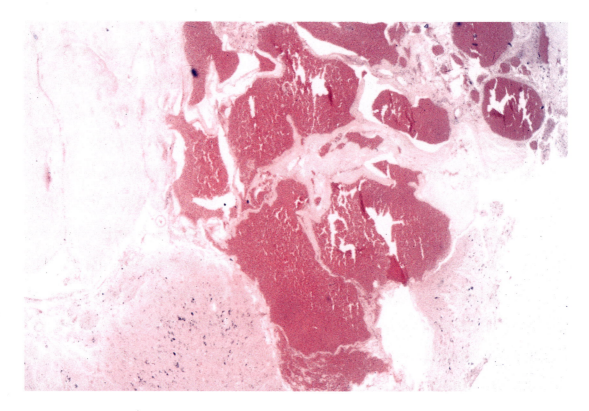

Figure 6.33 Cavernous hemangioma. Low-power view of the histology shows numerous large dilated venous channels in the leptomeninges on the surface of a temporal lobe, which shows gliosis, focal cavitation and hemosiderin discoloration. (H & E)

Table 6.13 Classification of lesions of the temporal lobe in intractable complex partial seizures. With permission from reference 9

(1) Ammon's horn sclerosis
  (a) Classical
  (b) End folium

(2) Neoplastic lesions
  (a) Mixed tumors
    (i) Ganglioglioma
    (ii) Dysembryoplastic neuroepithelial tumor
    (iii) Mixed glial tumors
  (b) Gliomas

(3) Familial and metabolic diseases
  (a) With focal lesions; phakomatosis

(4) Malformative lesions
  (a) Cortical dysplasias
    (i) Focal cortical dysplasia
    (ii) Microdysgenesis
  (b) Vascular malformations
    (i) Arteriovenous malformations
    (ii) Cavernous malformations

(5) Cerebrovascular disease and trauma

(6) Inflammatory/infectious
  (a) Fulminant encephalitis, meningitis
  (b) Chronic encephalitis, meningitis
  (c) Rasmussen's 'encephalitis'

(7) Non-specific lesions

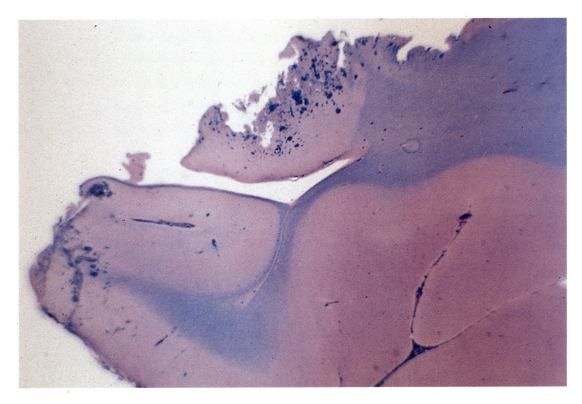

Figure 6.34 Mesial temporal sclerosis. Histological view of a temporal lobectomy shows the hippocampus to be shrunken and discolored. (H & E–luxol fast blue)

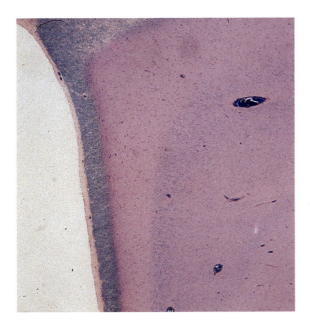

Figure 6.35 Mesial temporal sclerosis. Higher-power view of the CA1 sector of Figure 6.36 reveals the complete absence of neurons and the presence of isomorphous gliosis. (H & E–luxol fast blue)

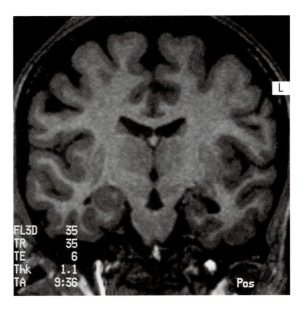

Figure 6.36 Left hippocampal atrophy. A right-handed woman had experienced prolonged 'febrile' convulsions in association with otitis media at the age of 18 months and refractory complex partial seizures from early childhood. Wada testing revealed right cerebral dominance and impaired left-hemisphere memory function. T1-weighted coronal MRI demonstrates marked hippocampal asymmetry with atrophy of the left side associated with a dilated temporal horn of the left lateral ventricle

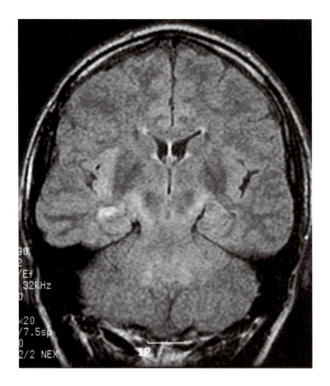

Figure 6.37 Right hippocampal sclerosis. A 26-year-old man with a history of febrile convulsions until the age of 4 years, and refractory complex partial seizures from the age of 12. MRI shows right hippocampal atrophy with high signal on FLAIR imaging

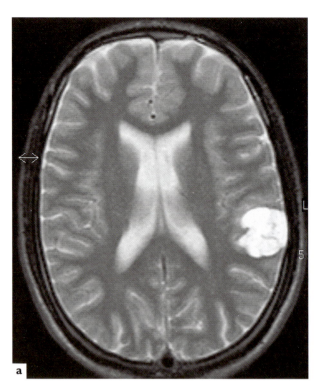

a

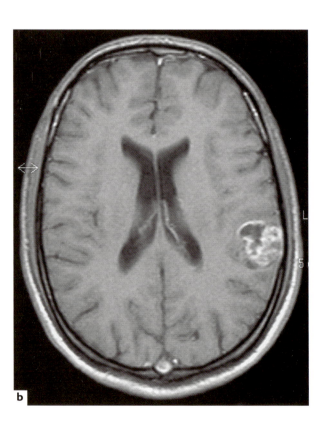

b

Focal cortical dysplasia

Focal cortical dysplasia is the most common developmental disorder causing epilepsy. Although extratemporal lesions predominate, this pathology is reported in 6–20% of cases of temporal lobe epilepsy. The lesions are highly epileptogenic, causing refractory epilepsy in up to 90% of patients; a history of status epilepticus (occurring in childhood), is obtainable in up to one-third of cases.

MRI (Figures 6.43 and 6.44) reveals focal areas of cortical thickening, poor gray–white matter differentiation and shallow sulci. A spectrum of pathology has been identified (Figures 6.45 and 6.46), ranging from mild cortical disorganization to lesions displaying abnormalities of neuronal migration, cellular division and differentiation. The outcome of surgery depends on the extent of resection, degree of dysplasia and postexcisional EEG appearances. Temporal lobe lesions have a more favorable outcome.

Figure 6.38 Ganglioglioma. A 30-year-old woman presented with tonic-clonic seizures, preceded by a brief aura of a tingling in her right arm. MRI shows a 2 cm cortically based lesion in the left parietal lobe. Histology showed this to be a ganglioglioma

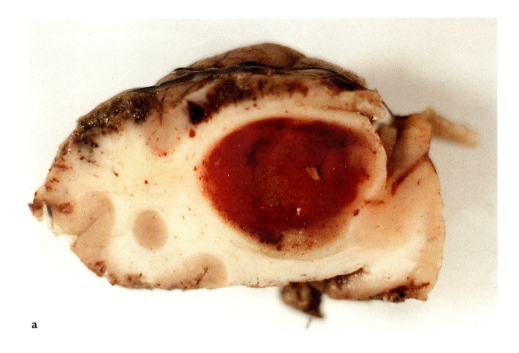

a

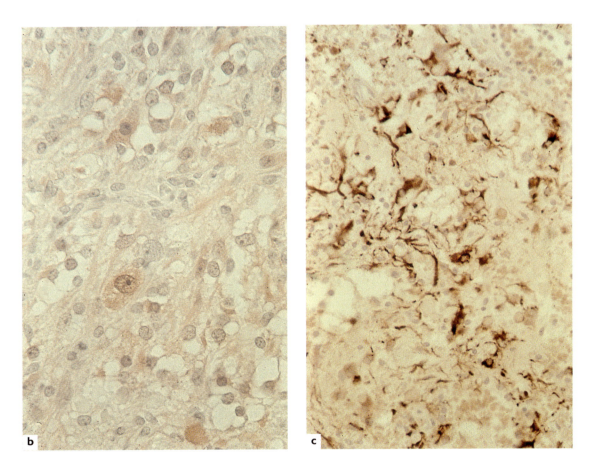

b   c

Figure 6.39 Ganglioglioma. This resected temporal lobe shows a well-circumscribed tumor (a); these are the typical appearances and location for a ganglioglioma. Immunocytochemistry of the histology for protein gene product (PGP) 9.5 (b) shows several positive-staining well-differentiated neoplastic neurons and processes within a glial background. Immunocytochemistry of the histology for glial fibrillary acidic protein (c) reveals the presence of neurons with positive-staining astrocytes. These are an integral constituent of the lesion, but it is not always clear whether or not they are neoplastic

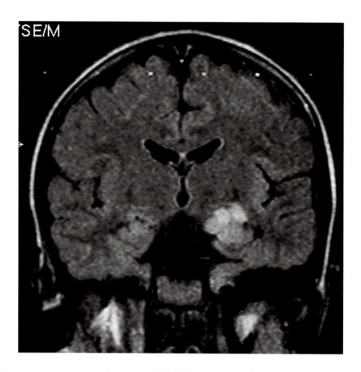

Figure 6.40 Dysembryoplastic neuroepithelial tumor (DNET) or low-grade tumor. A 12-year-old boy with a 12-month history of two partial and one secondarily generalized tonic-clonic seizures. An initial interictal EEG was normal, a repeat sleep-deprived EEG (recorded for 1 hour) demonstrated two brief left temporal discharges – axial, FLAIR MRI demonstrates a lesion in the medial part of the left temporal lobe with high signal within the lesion; on T1-weighted images the lesion was hypointense in comparison with normal gray matter. There was no enhancement after intravenous gadolinium. Two further MRI scans undertaken 12 and 24 months later showed no change in the size or signal characteristics of the lesion. A biopsy of the lesion has not been undertaken. The patient has been seizure-free for 22 months on levetiracetam monotherapy

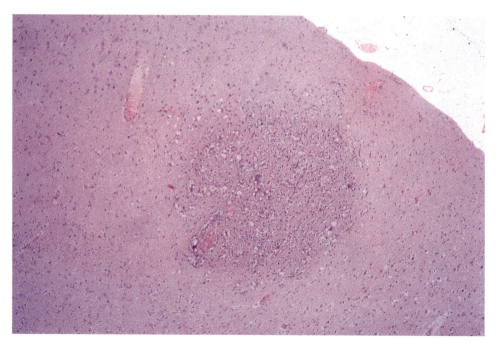

Figure 6.41 Dysembryoplastic neuroepithelial tumor (DNET). Histology of the cerebral cortex shows the characteristically nodular and intracortical architecture of the lesion. (H & E)

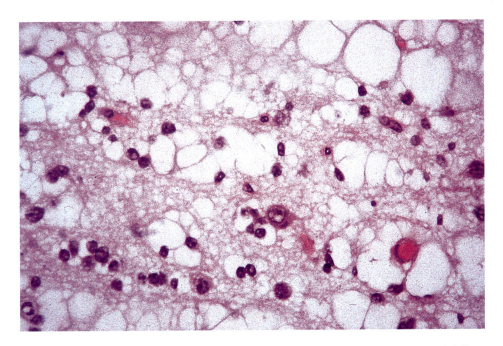

Figure 6.42 Dysembryoplastic neuroepithelial tumor. High-power view of Figure 6.43 shows well-differentiated neurons and glial cells floating in an extracellular matrix. These lesions are biologically indolent and probably hamartomatous. (H & E)

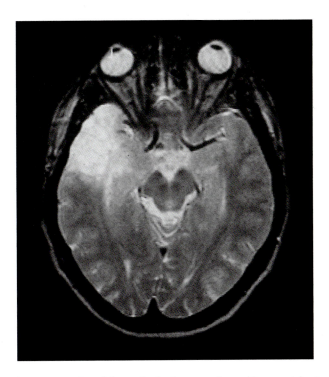

Figure 6.43 Focal cortical dysplasia. A 23-year-old man had a history of complex partial seizures from the age of 12 years. Wada testing demonstrated defective memory function on the right side. MRI shows an area of hyperintensity involving the anterior and lateral aspects of the right temporal lobe. He remains completely seizure free 1 year after a right anterior temporal lobectomy

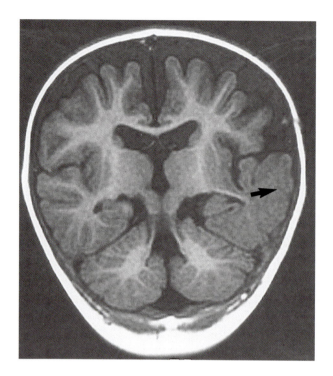

Figure 6.44 Focal cortical dysplasia. A 9-year-old girl with a 6-year history of frequent partial and infrequent secondarily generalized tonic-clonic seizures; she has global developmental delay (particularly affecting speech and language). Coronal, T1-weighted MRI demonstrates a thickened and dysplastic left temporal lobe with no white–gray matter differentiation and crude gyral formation (arrow). Both the ventricular and extra-ventricular spaces are increased, particularly around the left cerebral hemisphere

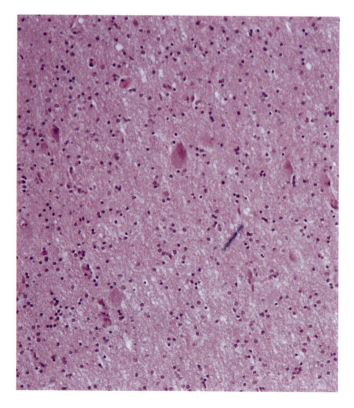

Figure 6.45 Focal cortical dysplasia. Histology of the cerebral cortex shows disordered architecture with abnormal neurons, some of which are situated in the subcortical white matter. (H & E)

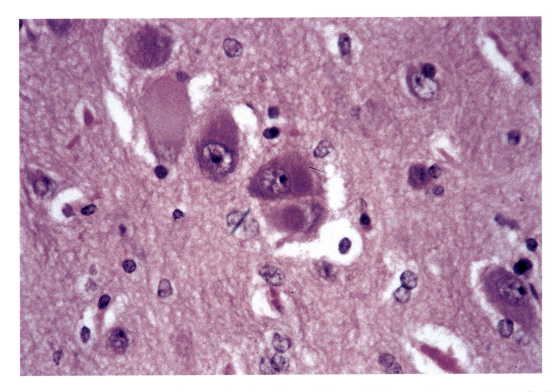

Figure 6.46 Focal cortical dysplasia. High-power histological view of the cerebral cortex shows morphologically abnormal neurons containing inclusions of cytoskeletal and other subcellular material. (H & E)

Malformations

These are characterized by disorganization of the cytoarchitecture of the brain or its vessels. Microdysgenesis is not visible radiologically, but has recently been described in isolation and in association with other pathology in patients with temporal lobe epilepsy and in patients with generalized epilepsy, particularly in the frontal lobes. Thus, an independent etiological role in focal epilepsy has not been defined. Vascular and arteriovenous malformations, and cavernous angiomas account for 2–10% of cases in reported series. Cavernomas may be familial and multiple.

Miscellaneous

Strokes, head trauma, meningitis and encephalitis rarely cause single focal resectable lesions. Post-traumatic cerebral contusion and focal scarring as a consequence of cerebral abscess account for a small proportion of surgical cases. Non-specific pathology has been reported in 20–30% of a number of a large series of patients, and is consistently associated with the poorest outcome. However, careful presurgical selection and improved operative techniques have reduced the incidence of negative histology in recent reports.

DUAL PATHOLOGY

With the continuing development of sophisticated neuroimaging modalities (both structural and functional), a number of patients with intractable (predominantly partial) epilepsy have been found to have evidence of dual pathology – hippocampal atrophy or mesial temporal sclerosis and another lesion[11]. The most frequently encountered 'other' lesions include a neuronal migration disorder (usually malformations of cortical development or cortical dysplasia) and porencephalic cysts. Less common 'other' lesions include low-grade tumors, vascular malformations and periventricular leukomalacia.

Dual pathology is seen in patients of all ages, including young children (Figure 6.47). The precise etiology and relationship of the two pathologies are as yet unclear, but it is possible that they share a

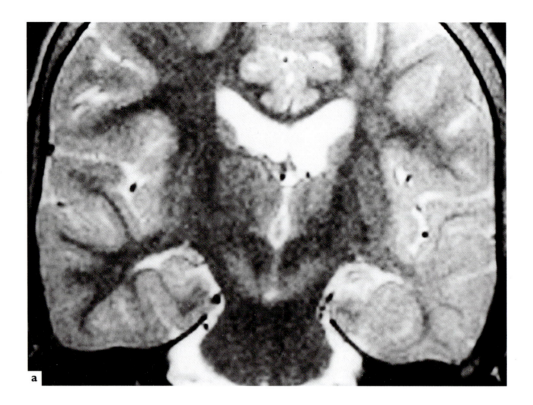

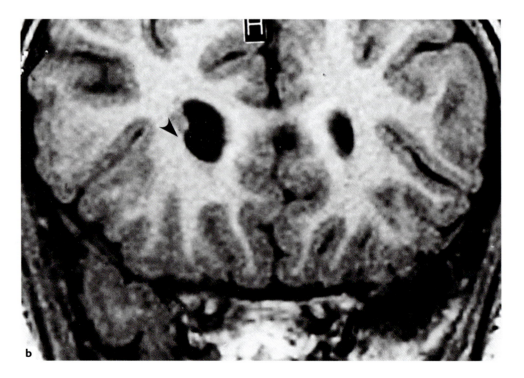

Figure 6.47 Dual pathology. An 11-year-old girl had a 4-year history of poorly controlled complex partial seizures (with predominantly temporal lobe symptomatology), and no history of 'febrile convulsions' and no cutaneous or radiological stigmata (or family history) of tuberous sclerosis. T2-weighted coronal MRI shows hippocampal sclerosis in the left temporal lobe (a) and subependymal heterotopic gray matter adjacent to, and indenting, the frontal horn of the right lateral ventricle (arrowed) (b). EEG showed only a left temporal slow-wave discharge

common pathogenetic mechanism with onset during pre- or perinatal development[12].

Alternatively, one may have caused the other. The extratemporal lesion (for example, cortical dysplasia) may be responsible for initiating early-onset, frequent, repeated and prolonged seizures (with or without associated febrile illness) which consequently cause, or at least contribute to, the mesial temporal sclerosis.

Dual pathology is clearly an important phenomenon requiring further clarification, as it has significant implications when planning surgical treatment for lesional epilepsy[12].

REFERENCES

1. Mackay MT, Weiss SK, Adams-Weber T, et al. Pracaport of the American Academy of Neurology and the Child Neurology Society. Neurology 2004; 62: 1668–81

2. Pennell PB. Using current evidence in selecting antiepileptic drugs for use during pregnancy. Curr Rev Clin Sci 2005; 5: 45–51

3. Scottish Intercollegiate Guidelines Network. Diagnosis and management of epilepsy. www.sign.ac.uk/pdf/sign70.pdf (accessed December 2004)

4. National Institute for Clinical Excellence. The epilepsies: diagnosis and management of the epilepsies in children and young people in primary and secondary care. www.nice.org.uk/CG020NICEguideline (accessed 2005)

5. The Status Epilepticus Working Party. The treatment of convulsive status epilepticus in children. Arch Dis Child 2000; 83: 413–19

6. McIntyre J, Robertson S, Norris E, et al. Safety and efficacy of buccal midazolam versus rectal diazepam for emergency treatment of seizures in children: a randomized controlled trial. Lancet 2005; 366: 205–10

7. Boon P, Vonck K, De Reuck J, Caemaert J. Vagus nerve stimulation for refractory epilepsy. Seizure 2001; 10: 448–55

8. Wheless JW, Baumgartner J. Vagal nerve stimulation therapy. Drugs Today 2004; 40: 501–15

9. Goodman, JH. Brain stimulation as a therapy for epilepsy. Adv Exp Med Biol 2004; 548: 239–47

10. Engel J Jr, ed. Surgical Treatment of the Epilepsies. New York: Raven Press, 1993

11. Cendes F, Cook MJ, Watson C, et al. Frequency and characteristics of dual pathology in patients with lesional epilepsy. Neurology 1995; 45: 2058–64

12. Wyllie E, Comair Y, Ruggieri P, et al. Epilepsy surgery in the setting of periventricular leukomalacia and focal cortical dysplasia. Neurology 1996; 46: 839–41

Index